Advances in Dosimetry and New Trends in Radiopharmaceuticals

Edited by Otolorin Adelaja Osibote and Elisabeth Eppard

Published in London, United Kingdom

Advances in Dosimetry and New Trends in Radiopharmaceuticals
http://dx.doi.org/10.5772/intechopen.110965
Edited by Otolorin Adelaja Osibote and Elisabeth Eppard

Contributors
E. Ishmael Parsai, Ebrahim Delpasand, Elahheh Salari, Elisabeth Eppard, Ethel Velásquez, Eóin N. Molloy, Foteini Simopoulou, Fran Laurie, Fred Prior, George Kyrgias, Hojjat Ahmadzadehfar, Joel Saltz, Kiki Theodorou, Koren Smith, Linda Ding, Mark Rosen, Maryann Bishop-Jodoin, Matt Iandoli, Michael Knopp, Mohsen Bakhshi Kashi, Nasim Vahidfar, Otolorin Adelaja Osibote, Panagiotis Iliopoulos, Peyman Sheikhzadeh, Roberto Mercado, Saeed Afshar, Saeed Farzanefar, Silvia Lagos, Siroos Mirzaei, Stephen Kry, Thomas J. FitzGerald, Vasileios Simopoulos, Yalda Salehi, Ying Xiao

First published in London, United Kingdom, 2024 by IntechOpen
IntechOpen is the global imprint of INTECHOPEN LIMITED, registered in England and Wales, registration number: 11086078, 5 Princes Gate Court, London, SW7 2QJ, United Kingdom

British Library Cataloguing-in-Publication Data
A catalogue record for this book is available from the British Library

Additional hard and PDF copies can be obtained from orders@intechopen.com

Advances in Dosimetry and New Trends in Radiopharmaceuticals
Edited by Otolorin Adelaja Osibote and Elisabeth Eppard
p. cm.
Print ISBN 978-0-85466-008-7
Online ISBN 978-0-85466-007-0
eBook (PDF) ISBN 978-0-85466-009-4

For EU product safety concerns:
IN TECH d.o.o., Prolaz Marije Krucifikse Kozulić 3, 51000 Rijeka, Croatia,
info@intechopen.com or visit our website at intechopen.com.

Meet the editors

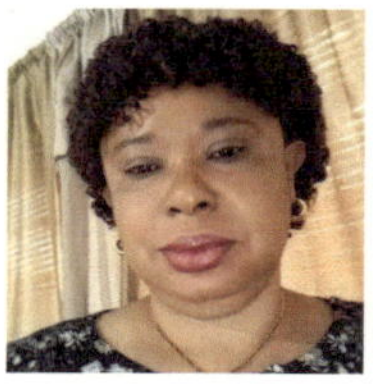

Otolorin Adelaja Osibote is a Senior Lecturer of Medical and Health Physics in the Department of Mathematics and Physics, Faculty of Applied Sciences, Cape Peninsula University of Technology, South Africa, where she teaches subjects in physics. She graduated with a second-class upper in Physics (Hons) and an MSc in Engineering Physics (Medical and Health Physics). She received a DSc in Public Health (Medical Physics) from Escola Nacional de Saude Publica, FIOCRUZ, Brazil. She has authored about eighty papers in international journals and international conference proceedings. She has been involved in several research projects funded by her institution. She is a reviewer for several international scientific journals. Her research interests include irradiation and radioactivity contents of some foodstuffs, dosimetry studies in diagnostic radiology, radiation protection and safety, and assessment of metal contents in environmental samples.

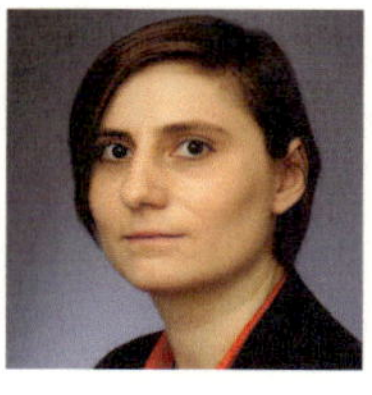

Dr. Elisabeth Eppard is a radiochemist working on the development and process implementation of new compounds for theranostic application. In 2013, she obtained her Ph.D. under Prof. Rösch at the Institute of Nuclear Chemistry, Johannes Gutenberg University Mainz, Germany, where she worked on radiometal-based radiopharmaceuticals. After four years as a junior research group leader in the Department of Nuclear Medicine, University Hospital Bonn, Germany, Dr. Eppard joined Positronpharma SA, Santiago, Chile, as a senior scientist in 2018. There, she was responsible for research and clinical applications based on 68Ga-, 44Sc-, and 177Lu-labeled theranostics. Since 2021, she has been a radiochemist in the Department of Nuclear Medicine, University Hospital Magdeburg, Germany, where she is continuing her research.

Contents

Preface **IX**

Section 1
Advances in Dosimetry **1**

Chapter 1 **3**
Introductory Chapter: Dosimetry in Radiopharmacy
by Otolorin Adelaja Osibote and Elisabeth Eppard

Chapter 2 **7**
Advances in Radiotherapy Dosimetry Techniques and Pre-Treatment Verification
by Elahheh Salari and E. Ishmael Parsai

Chapter 3 **39**
Modern Dosimetry in Radiation Oncology Clinical Trials
by Koren Smith, Linda Ding, Maryann Bishop-Jodoin, Matt Iandoli, Fran Laurie, Stephen Kry, Michael Knopp, Mark Rosen, Ying Xiao, Fred Prior, Joel Saltz and Thomas J. FitzGerald

Chapter 4 **53**
Review on Cone Beam Computed Tomography (CBCT) Dose in Patients Undergoing Image Guided Radiotherapy (IGRT)
by Panagiotis Iliopoulos, Foteini Simopoulou, Vasileios Simopoulos, George Kyrgias and Kiki Theodorou

Section 2
New Trends in Radiopharmaceuticals **73**

Chapter 5 **75**
Recent Advances of Copper-64 Based Radiopharmaceuticals in Nuclear Medicine
by Nasim Vahidfar, Mohsen Bakhshi Kashi, Saeed Afshar, Peyman Sheikhzadeh, Saeed Farzanefar, Yalda Salehi, Ebrahim Delpasand, Eóin N. Molloy, Siroos Mirzaei, Hojjat Ahmadzadehfar and Elisabeth Eppard

Chapter 6 **99**
Radiochemical Purity and Identity in Radiopharmaceuticals: Design and Improvement of Quality Control Methods by HPLC
by Roberto Mercado, Silvia Lagos and Ethel Velásquez

Preface

This book provides comprehensive details on the advances in dosimetry in radiotherapy for effective and efficient treatment, reducing patient risks. This book is organized into two sections: "Advances in Dosimetry" and "New Trends in Radiopharmaceuticals". The first section covers different dosimetry methods that are used in radiotherapy systems, such as image-guided radiotherapy (IGRT). The second section covers the types and quality of radiochemical applications in nuclear medicine and their radiation dosimetry analysis.

Otolorin Adelaja Osibote
Faculty of Applied Science,
Department of Mathematics and Physics,
Cape Peninsula University of Technology,
Cape Town, South Africa

Dr. Elisabeth Eppard
Department of Nuclear Medicine,
University Hospital Magdeburg,
Magdeburg, Germany

Section 1

Advances in Dosimetry

Chapter 1

Introductory Chapter: Dosimetry in Radiopharmacy

Otolorin Adelaja Osibote and Elisabeth Eppard

1. Introduction

Nuclear medicine and radiopharmacy are based on the scientific ideas and discoveries of the beginning of the last century and are decisively shaped by their respective discoverers. Among them are H. Becquerel, M. Curie & P. Curie (Nobel Prize 1903 "discovery of spontaneous radioactivity" and "researches on radiation phenomena…"), I. Curie & F. Joliot (Nobel Prize 1935 "synthesis of new radioactive elements"), G. de Hevesy (Nobel Prize 1943 "for the use of isotopes as tracers in the study of chemical processes"), O. Hahn, F. Strassmann, L. Meitner & O. R. Frisch (Nobel Prize 1944 only to O. Hahn "Discovery of the fission of heavy nuclei"), R. S. Yalow & S. A. Berson (Nobel Prize 1977 only to R. S. Yalow "Development of radioimmunoassays of peptide hormones") or Saul Hertz and Arthur Roberts [1, 2].

Based on their fundamental discoveries, the two closely intertwined disciplines developed further and established their place in the clinical routine. Today, radiopharmaceuticals are indispensable to clinical diagnosis and therapy for various diseases [1].

Growing experience in radiochemistry and its fusion with organic chemistry further facilitated the application of radionuclides and radiolabeled compounds in medicine. All this was accompanied by continuous technical development, driven by the natural sciences and industry, which provided the appropriate equipment and invaluable contributions from other disciplines such as mathematics, physics, and biology. In every respect, radiopharmacy or radiopharmaceutical chemistry is an excellent example of the interdisciplinary nature of modern science and technology.

Unnoticed by the general public, technetium-99 m, a radioisotope of a biologically irrelevant element, is used in millions of diagnostic procedures yearly. Various tracers are radiolabeled to cover a wide range of diagnostic applications. In addition, an ^{18}F-radiolabeled derivative of the most abundant monosaccharide, glucose, plays an essential role in quantifying glucose metabolism, which can indicate severe disease, although the derivative does not exist naturally.

The spectrum of available radiopharmaceuticals ranges from non-specific perfusion tracers to highly selective, targeted tracers suitable for various applications (both diagnostic and therapeutic). Some of these radiopharmaceuticals have been used in routine clinical use for decades. These include iodine- and technetium-labeled compounds. Highly specific, targeted tracers have become increasingly important over the past decade. Despite their relatively short history of routine use, their impact on nuclear medicine has been profound. This is particularly evident in the ever-increasing number of approved radiopharmaceuticals and clinical trials. Radiopharmacy and nuclear medicine are new growth markets [3]. Today, the influence of radiopharmaceutical chemistry extends far beyond supplying radiopharmaceuticals to nuclear medicine centers. It also plays a crucial role in industrial drug development and fundamental biochemical and medical research.

The development of radiopharmaceuticals is a complex, interdisciplinary process that depends on many factors. It begins with the selection of a suitable radionuclide. Its physical properties must match the type of application. For radiolabeling, its chemical properties must match those of the selected precursor. The radionuclide and the precursor must be available in the highest quality and quantity. During the reaction, the precursor must not be degraded or destroyed by the reaction conditions or the radiation to achieve acceptable (activity) yields. Pharmaceutical standards must be consistently maintained. In addition, the radioactive decay and half-life of the radionuclide determine every step of the process, from the start of radionuclide production to its final use in the patient. Transport, storage, and patient management are more complex and susceptible to disruption than traditional non-radioactive drugs. Nonetheless, nuclear medicine is an integral part of precision medicine, with an ever-increasing demand for radiopharmaceuticals in patient care.

The development, preclinical, and clinical evaluation of new radiopharmaceuticals involves the identification and targeted use of novel molecular targets for effective and efficient imaging and therapy. This includes binding modeling, biodistribution, pharmacokinetics, process optimization, (further) development of suitable manufacturing and quality control methods, and dosimetry studies. All this ultimately leads to an optimized, automated synthesis of pharmaceutical-grade radiopharmaceuticals.

Radiotherapy and radiopharmaceuticals aim to increase the life expectancy of cancer patients; however, this increase is accompanied by the risk of subsequent radiation-induced secondary cancers, which poses a significant challenge. To prevent a reduction in life expectancy, dosimetry is essential at various points in radiopharmaceutical therapy, from pre-treatment planning through the absorbed dose to the target organ or tumor to the total body dose.

Dosimetry studies in radiotherapy aim to calculate the dose absorbed by normal tissues and tumors and anticipate radiation's biological effects. Absorbed dose calculations take into account (patient-dependent) anatomy, radiopharmaceutical biodistribution, and (patient-independent) radionuclide properties [4]. Therefore, the role of medical physicists is to ensure the safety of patients undergoing radiotherapy by ensuring that the radiotherapy equipment is correctly calibrated and delivers accurate radiation.

Radiotherapy dosimetry methodologies must take into account the types of radionuclides, i.e., low (beta particles and photons) and high (alpha particles) linear energy transfer emitters, for effective treatment planning [5]. In conclusion, improvements in dosimetry studies will help develop new advances in radiotherapy for improved efficacy, leading to fewer complications.

Author details

Otolorin Adelaja Osibote[1*] and Elisabeth Eppard[2]

1 Department of Mathematics and Physics, Faculty of Applied Science, Cape Peninsula University of Technology, Cape Town, South Africa

2 Faculty of Medicine, University Clinic for Radiology and Nuclear Medicine, Otto von Guericke University (OvGU), Magdeburg, Germany

*Address all correspondence to: elisabeth.eppard@med.ovgu.de

References

[1] Baum RP, Rösch F. Theranostics, Gallium-68, and Other Radionuclides. A Pathway to Personalized Diagnosis and Treatment. Berlin, New York: Springer; 2013 (Recent results in cancer research, v.194)

[2] The Nobel Foundation. Hg. v. The Nobel Foundation. Online verfügbar unter: https://www.nobelprize.org/prizes/lists/all-nobel-prizes/1909-1901/ [zuletzt geprüft am Januar 25, 2024]

[3] Bodei L, Herrmann K, Schöder H, Scott AM, Lewis JS. Radiotheranostics in oncology: Current challenges and emerging opportunities. Nature Reviews Clinical Oncology. 2022;**19**(8):534-550. DOI: 10.1038/s41571-022-00652-y

[4] O'Donoghue J, Zanzonico P, Humm J, Kesner A. Dosimetry in radiopharmaceutical therapy. Journal of Nuclear Medicine: Official Publication, Society of Nuclear Medicine. 2022;**63**(10):1467-1474. DOI: 10.2967/jnumed.121.262305

[5] Sgouros G, Hobbs RF. Dosimetry for radiopharmaceutical therapy. Seminars in Nuclear Medicine. 2014;**44**(3):172-178. DOI: 10.1053/j.semnuclmed.2014.03.007

Chapter 2

Advances in Radiotherapy Dosimetry Techniques and Pre-Treatment Verification

Elahheh Salari and E. Ishmael Parsai

Abstract

In the fight against cancer, radiation therapy plays a vital role, with its two essential approaches: internal, involving the insertion or implantation of radioactive material into the patient's body, or uptake of radiopharmaceutical, and external. Precise delivery of the appropriate radiation dosage to the tumor is critical for achieving favorable outcomes. This is where dosimetry becomes crucial—a scientific discipline that involves measuring, calculating, and evaluating radiation doses. Medical physicists utilize dosimetry to ensure the accuracy and proper calibration of machines that administer ionizing radiation, ensuring safety. This chapter provides a brief overview of advanced techniques and equipment used in dosimetry, with a primary focus on photon and electron dosimetry, the most widely employed forms of radiation for radiotherapy worldwide.

Keywords: external beam dosimetry, *in-vivo* dosimetry, detectors, phantoms, patient-specific QA

1. Introduction

Radiotherapy aims to deliver a specific amount of radiation to the tumor while minimizing damage to nearby organs at risk (OAR). Over the past decade, there has been a surge in the development of advanced radiotherapy techniques in both computation of radiation dose (inverse planning) and delivery techniques such as Intensity Modulated Radiation Therapy (IMRT) and volumetric modulated arc therapy (VMAT). The main objective of these sophisticated developments is mainly to enhance target dose uniformity and minimize high-dose regions and doses to nearby tissues and organs-at-risk (OARs). These advanced techniques are more complicated than 3D conformal therapy and require sophisticated tools and techniques for dosimetry to guarantee that the delivered dose corresponds accurately with the planned doses. Numerous guidelines and dosimeter devices, including detectors, phantoms, and electronic devices, have been designed for this purpose. This chapter will discuss the various equipment and methods used for dosimetry in photon and electron therapies, brachytherapy, neutron, and proton therapies.

2. Dosimetry of photon and electron beams

2.1 Summary of AAPM task group 51

In radiotherapy, the American Association of Physicists in Medicine Task Group 51 (AAPM TG-51) [1] and its Addendum [2] are one of the main dosimetry references for external high-energy photon and electron beams. These guidelines are based on measurements conducted with **ionization chambers (IC)**, the most common radiotherapy radiation detectors. These detectors are made up of a gas-filled chamber that has two electrodes of opposing polarity, namely, the anode and cathode. The electrodes can be in the form of either parallel plates (known as plane-parallel IC) or a cylinder (thimble) with an internal anode wire located coaxially. Ionization chambers are a type of detector that collects ion pairs from gases to measure incident radiation [3, 4]. By creating an electric field in the gas-filled cavity through a voltage potential applied between electrodes, charged particles move to electrodes of opposite polarity. This generates an ionization current, which is measured by an electrometer circuit. The current ranges from femtoamperes to picoamperes, proportional to the radiation dose, and depends on the chamber design [3]. Cylindrical chambers are frequently used in Ref. dosimetry applications of MV photon beams and electron beams (>10 MeV), while plane-parallel is designed for low energy electrons (<10 MeV) as well as in applications where precise measurement location is important such as measurement of electron percent depth dose distributions [1].

An ion chamber is calibrated in terms of absorbed dose-to-water in a standard laboratory's reference quality Co^{60} gamma-ray beam. The calibration is valid under reference conditions, which specify a field size of 10×10 cm^2 and a reference depth of 10 cm under the water surface for photon beams [5]. For electron beams, the reference depth is determined by Eq. (1)

$$D_{ref} = 0.6R_{50} - 0.1\ \text{cm} \tag{1}$$

where R_{50} is the depth at which ionization drops to 50% of its maximum value. The reference field size is 10×10 cm^2 and 20×20 cm^2 where $R_{50} \leq 8.5$ cm and $R_{50} >$ 8.5 cm, respectively.

The absorbed dose in water is calculated by a general formalism for both photon and electron beams Eq. (2).

$$D_w^Q = MN_{D,w}^Q (Gy) \tag{2}$$

where M is the fully corrected reading of the electrometer, which is expressed in units of C or rdg, and can be calculated using Eq. (3)

$$M = P_{ion}P_{TP}P_{pol}P_{elec}M_{raw}(C\ or\ rdg) \tag{3}$$

P_{ion} corrects the incomplete ion collection efficiency of the detector, and its value should be ≤1.05. There are two formulas to consider when dealing with continuous beams, such as Co-60 (Eq. 4), and pulsed or pulsed-swept beams (Eq. 5):

$$P_{ion} = \frac{1.00 - \left(\frac{V_H}{V_L}\right)^2}{\frac{M_{raw}^H}{M_{raw}^L} \times \left(\frac{V_H}{V_L}\right)^2} \tag{4}$$

and

$$P_{ion} = \frac{1.00 - \frac{V_H}{V_L}}{\frac{M_{raw}^H}{M_{raw}^L} \times \frac{V_H}{V_L}} \tag{5}$$

V_H is the standard operating voltage for the ion chamber, and M_{raw}^H is the raw reading at this voltage.

V_L is reduced voltage (at least half of V_H), and M_{raw}^L is the raw reading of the detector at the corresponding voltage.

P_{TP} is the temperature–pressure correction factor since calibration factors are given for standard environmental conditions of T_0 = 22°C and P_0 = 101.33 kPa (1 atmosphere).

$$P_{TP} = \frac{273.2 + T}{273.2 + 22} \times \frac{101.3}{P} \tag{6}$$

P_{pol} corrects the polarity effects and depends on beam quality and other conditions such as cable position. To ensure an accurate calibration procedure, it's essential to apply this correction every time.

$$P_{pol} = \left| \frac{M_{raw}^+ - M_{raw}^-}{2M_{raw}} \right| \tag{7}$$

The raw readings for positive and negative normal operating voltage of the detector are represented by M_{raw}^+ and M_{raw}^-, respectively, and M_{raw} can be either M_{raw}^+ or M_{raw}^-.

It is recommended that the polarity correction be kept below 0.3%, although the Addendum to TG-51 permits up to 0.4%.

P_{elec} is the electrometer correction factor when performing separate calibrations for the electrometer and ion chamber. It is advisable to calibrate both the ion chamber and the electrometer together, in this case, P_{elec} = 1.00. Moreover, this factor has a unity value for cross-calibrated parallel plate chambers as it cancels out of the final equations (section X C of TG-51).

$N_{D,w}^Q$ is the absorbed dose to water calibration factor for the user's ion chamber located in an arbitrary beam of quality Q, under reference conditions, and its value can be expressed in units of Gy/C or Gy/rdg. Typically, absorbed-dose calibration factors are obtained under reference conditions using a Co-60 beam. In this case, $N_{D,w}^Q$ is calculated for the beam of quality Q, which can be photon or electron using Eq. (8).

$$N_{D,w}^Q = k_Q N_{D,w}^{60\ Co} \tag{8}$$

k_Q is the quality conversion factor that converts the absorbed dose to water calibration factor for a ^{60}Co beam into the calibration factor for a beam of quality Q. This factor is chamber specific for photon beams and its value for most ion chambers used as reference chamber can be found in section IX.B of TG-51.

For electron beams, the quality conversion factor has two components (Eq. 9):

$$k_Q = P_{gr}^Q k_{R50} \tag{9}$$

where P_{gr}^{Q} is one for plane-parallel chambers and only applies to the cylindrical ion chamber and corrects for the ionization gradient at the reference depth. To determine this factor, the user must follow the measuring procedure outlined in TG-51. k_{R50} that has two components as follows (Eq. 10).

$$k_{R50} = k'_{R50} k_{ecal} \tag{10}$$

k_{ecal} is the photon-electron conversion factor specified for each individual ion chamber in TG-51.

k'_{R50} is the electron beam quality conversion factor and depends on the beam quality.

In an electron beam, the dose of water is given by:

$$D_{w}^{Q} = MP_{gr}^{Q} k'_{R50} k_{ecal} N_{D,w}^{60Co}\ (Gy) \tag{11}$$

To prevent any complications with additional waterproof sleeves and potential air gaps, it is best to use a waterproof ion chamber. An additional waterproofing sleeve is necessary if the chamber is not waterproof. A waterproofing sleeve should reduce the air gaps near the chamber wall ($\leq$ 0.2 mm) and should be made of polymethyl-methacrylate (PMMA) $\leq$ 1 mm thick.

Clinical reference measurements must be performed in a water phantom with a minimum size of 30 $\times$ 30 $\times$ 30 cm^3, and the use of non-water phantoms is not allowed. If the beam penetrates the plastic wall of the water phantom and the wall's thickness exceeds 0.2 cm, it is necessary to adjust all depths to their water equivalent values. This is achieved by measuring from the outer surface of the wall when the phantom contains water while also considering the density of the wall.

The beam quality must be specified to determine the correct value of the quality conversion factor for electron and photon beams. Beam quality is characterized by a parameter related to the central-axis depth-dose curves for the beam.

For photon beams, it is the percentage depth dose at 10 cm depth in the water of 10x10 cm^2 open field size at SSD = 100 cm. If the energy of the photon beam is less than 10 MV (%dd(10) <75%), the value of %dd(10) is $\%dd(10)_X$. However, for beam energies >10 MV and flattening filter-free (FFF) beams, due to electron contamination, the value of $\%dd(10)_X$ is obtained from $\%dd(10)_{pb}$ parameter when the 1 mm thick lead foil is placed at the 50 $\pm$ 5 cm from a phantom surface:

$$\%dd(10)_x = \left[0.8905 + 0.00150\%dd(10)_{pb}\right]\%dd(10)_{pb} \tag{12}$$

And if the lead foil is located at 30 $\pm$ 1 cm above the phantom surface, $\%dd(10)_x$ is calculated by Eq. (13):

$$\%dd(10)_x = \left[0.8116 + 0.00264\%dd(10)_{pb}\right]\%dd(10)_{pb} \tag{13}$$

Moreover, if the $\%dd\ (10)_{pb}$ is less than 73 and 71% where the foil is at 50 and 30 cm, respectively, then $\%dd(10)_x = \%dd(10)_{pb}$.

It is important to use an SSD of 100 cm when determining the beam quality for photon and electron beams, as both %dd(10) and R_{50} are SSD dependent.

In the process of measurement, cylindrical and spherical chambers should be shifted to the effective point of measurement. The effective point is located upstream of the actual point of measurement. This is because the secondary electrons tend to move forward, causing a shift in the depth-dose curve toward shallower depths. Therefore, the upstream shift for **cylindrical** and **spherical chambers** is $0.6r_{cav}$ and $0.5r_{cav}$ for photon and electron beams, respectively, where r_{cav} is the radius of the ion chamber's cavity. No shift is required for **parallel plate chambers**, as the point of measurement is the center of the front (upstream) face of the chamber air cavity.

In summary, TG-51 applies to photon beams with an energy range of Co-60 to 50 MV and electron beams with nominal energies between 4 and 50 MeV and provides the following information: (1) Prescribing a methodology for clinical reference dosimetry, (2) determining the beam quality conversion factor for both photon and electron beams, (3) measuring gradient correction factor for cylindrical chambers in electron beams, (4) measuring various correction factors to correct the raw charge reading of the ion chamber, and (5) using cylindrical and plane-parallel ICs for absolute calibration measurements.

2.2 Detectors for patient-specific quality assurance

Intensity-modulated radiotherapy (IMRT) and VMAT treatment techniques involve many challenges, particularly the dosimetry of small fields, varying dose rates, low MU segments, multileaf collimator (MLC) motions, and gantry speed variations for VMAT [6, 7]. Furthermore, dosimetry conditions for IMRT/VMAT are significantly different from the open field conditions for which the chambers are calibrated. It is highly recommended to perform patient-specific quality assurance (QA) to identify any disagreements between the dose calculated by the treatment planning system (TPS) and the actual dose delivered by the treatment machine [8]. The patient-specific QA includes several dosimetric tasks that are performed before the treatment. Several phantoms and detectors such as cylindrical ion chambers, detector arrays, Gafchromic films, and so on have been designed and implemented for this purpose. To ensure accurate pre-treatment verifications, it is important to have a comprehensive understanding of detector/phantom characteristics, including energy and dose rate dependence, collecting volume size, charge leakage, design, and materials [9, 10].

2.2.1 Ionization chambers

In pre-treatment verification or patient-specific QA of IMRT treatment plans, a phantom (either 2D or 3D) is typically used to check the dose distribution, while an ion chamber is utilized for absolute dose verifications. As the plan becomes more complex, smaller field sizes and higher MU are required to achieve a conformal dose distribution. IMRT/VMAT plans include small control points or segments with a size of less than or equal to 1x1 cm^2. Therefore, for absolute dose verifications, it is recommended to use ion chambers with a small volume of 0.1 cc or less [11]. Nonetheless, there are potential downsides to using small ion chambers as their sensitivity may decrease with decreasing volume [6, 9, 12]. Leybovich et al. [9] evaluated the performance of ion chambers of varying volumes such as Farmer type NE 2581 0.6 cm^3 (NE Technology, Essex, UK), Capintec PR-06 0.6 cm^3 (Capintec, Inc., Ramsey, NJ), PTW 0.125 cm^3 (PTW-New York, Hicksville, NY), and Exradin A1 0.009 cm^3 (Standard Imaging Inc., Middleton, WI) for the absolute dose verification of tomographic and step-and-shoot IMRT treatment plans. Their study revealed that the response of 0.6 cc chambers was higher than the calculated dose when the chamber was partially irradiated. Additionally, the measurements from the smaller chambers (0.125 and 0.009 cm^3) required correction for charge leakage due to chamber sensitivity being proportional to volume [9]. Another study compared three different cylindrical chambers including a 0.015 cm^3 PTW-Freiburg 31,006 pinpoint (PTW-Freiburg, Freiburg, Germany), a 0.13 cm^3 Wellhöfer IC10 (Scanditronix Wellhöfer North America, Bartlett, TN), and a 0.69 cm^3 Farmer-type (FT) IC model NE2571 (Nuclear Enterprises, Fairfield, NJ) [6]. Their study indicated small ion chambers overresponded when irradiated with a small number of monitor units (MU) because the smallest-volume chambers are more sensitive to leakage compared to large-volume ion chambers. Evaluation of 50 IMRT treatment plan quality assurance procedures indicated the Farmer chamber measurements were found to be the closest to the TPS calculated values. However, all chambers measured higher doses than those predicted by TPS [6]. Research conducted by Kumar et al. [12] assessed the response of five different IC-phantom combinations in RapidArc therapy. This study included a Medtec IMRT phantom with Exradin (A16) micro-ion chamber (0.007 cm^3) and PTW pinpoint chamber (TM31014–0193) (0.015 cm^3), PTW-Octavius phantom with semiflex chamber (TM31010–1571) (0.125 cm^3) and PTW 2D-array 729 (T10024) (0.125 cm^3), and an indigenously made circular wax phantom with a 0.61 cm^3 chamber (NE 2571). All absolute dose measurements taken at the isocenter were compared to those calculated by the Eclipse TPS (Varian Medical Systems, Palo Alto, CA) version 8.6. The results showed that the leakage has a greater effect on small-volume chambers as the sensitivity of the chamber is directly related to its volume. Additionally, positioning is a very important factor when using smaller-volume chambers because they are more susceptible to errors caused by geometrical variations within the treatment fields (**Figure 1**) [12].

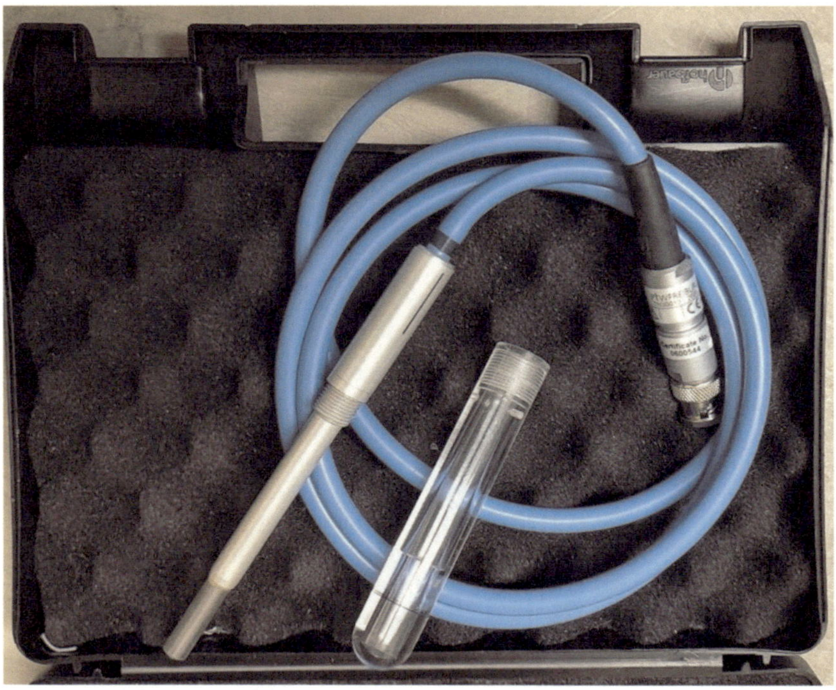

Figure 1.
Farmer chamber.

2.2.2 Gafchromic films

As aforementioned, verifying the accuracy of IMRT/VMAT delivery can be difficult due to numerous small fields, irregularities, steep dose gradients, and sharp penumbra. Consequently, the conventional method of measuring point doses using an IC for patient-specific QA is insufficient for highly modulated treatment fields like stereotactic radiosurgery (SRS) or Stereotactic Body Radiation Therapy (SBRT) where small targets are irradiated in a single fraction using a high-intensity photon beam [13]. Radiochromic films, typically referred to as "GAFChromic," with the added advantage of self-development have been employed for this purpose. Due to their high spatial resolution, they can provide a more accurate map of dose distribution in the sharp dose gradient regions [14]. GAFChromic™ EBT3 film is a radiochromic film produced by International Specialty Products Ashland Inc. (Covington, KY) for clinical dosimetry in 2011. The EBT3 film is very similar in dosimetric performance to previous generation EBT2 but has two major improvements: (1) the symmetric configuration of EBT3 eliminates measurement orientation effects and (2) the EBT3 prevents the formation of Newton rings that usually formed during film scanning [15, 16]. According to the manufacture documents [17], EBT3 film is made by laminating an active layer (28 μm) sandwiched between two identical polyester layers (125 μm each), which makes it more robust and allows water immersion. It is important to note that these films are sensitive to temperature and should be stored in an environment with a temperature below 25°C. It is crucial to avoid exposing them to temperatures above 50 degrees Celsius to ensure their quality and longevity [17, 18]. Several studies have been conducted on Gafchromic film characteristics, demonstrating they are energy- and dose-rate independent [19–22]. In particular, Sipilä et al. [21] measured the response of EBT3 films to photon (6 MV) and electron beams (6 to 16 MeV) and showed the energy dependence of EBT3 film is uniform within 0.5% across all electron beams. Including the 6 MV and the range of electron energies, the energy dependence of the EBT3 is about 1.1%, making it suitable for dosimetry of mixed photon/electron dose distributions [21]. One of the primary uses of EBT3 is for IMRT/VMAT verification, and multiple studies have indicated that these films are effective tools for this purpose [14, 16, 23]. The gamma index is widely used to compare the 2D/3D dose distribution calculated by TPS with the measured dose. This index compares the measured dose (evaluated dose distribution) point-by-point to that calculated dose (reference dose distribution) based on a distance to agreement (DTA) and a dose difference (DD) criterion [24]. In 2020, the assessment of quality assurance of IMRT plans under a 0.35 Tesla MR guided radiotherapy using Gafchromic™ EBT3 was conducted by Gungor et al. [23]. This study included 70 patients who received treatment with the ViewRay MRIdian® Linac from September 2018 to June 2019. According to their findings, 91% of all the QA analyses demonstrated a passing rate greater than 95% even for a tolerance of 2%/2 mm (%DD/DTA). Based on their analysis, it was determined that EBT3 film dosimetry is a reliable tool for gamma analysis evaluation of treatment plans, even under the presence of a 0.35 Tesla magnetic field [23]. Nevertheless, EBT3 has an optimal range of 0.2 to 10 Gy, which limits its usability. EBT-XD Gafchromic films were developed in 2015, offering optimal performance in the 40–4000 cGy dose range to address this issue. Its design is very similar to EBT3 films, but its active layer thickness is 25 μm. These films are best suited for patient-specific QA of SRS/SBRT techniques where high doses of radiation are delivered to targets [17, 25–27].

Film dosimetry presents several advantages, notably its water equivalence and the absence of correction factors. Additionally, it offers structural flexibility, protection against water and moisture infiltration, and independence from irradiation angles, boasting high detection resolution. Nonetheless, film dosimetry comes with certain drawbacks, including variations in radiochromic film characteristics, saturation time, and reliance on lot batch consistency. Additionally, film dosimetry depends on landscape and portrait scan orientation, with limitations for peripheral scanner devices, scanning region calibration, and lateral effect. All these disadvantages introduce uncertainties in dosimetry [26–32]; therefore, one can conclude that film dosimetry may not be the primary option for conducting patient-specific QA.

2.2.3 Detector arrays

Several commercial detector arrays have been developed for performing patient-specific IMRT/VMAT QA. **Tables 1** and **2** provide lists of the available array detectors commonly utilized in clinical settings.

Detector Array	**MapCHECK2**	**MapCHECK3**	**SRS MapCHECK**	**ArcCHECK**
Type of Detector	SunPoint Diode	SunPoint 2 Diode	SunPoint 2 Diode	SunPoint Diode
Active Detector Area (mm^2)	0.8 × 0.8	0.48 × 0.48	0.48 × 0.48	0.8 × 0.8
Array Size (cm^2)	26 × 32	26 × 32	7.7 × 7.7	21 × 21
Detector Spacing	7.07 mm	7.07 mm	2.47 mm	10 mm
Number of Detectors	1527	1527	1013	1386
Update Frequency (ms)	50	50	50	50
Inherent Buildup (g/cm^2)	2	1.5	2.75	3.3
Array Geometry	Flat	Flat	Flat	Helical Grid

Table 1.
List of diode arrays manufactured by SUN NUCLEAR corporation [33].

Detector Array	**OCTAVIUS detector 729**	**OCTAVIUS detector 1500**	**OCTAVIUS detector 1600**	**OCTAVIUS 1000 SRS**
Type of Detector	vented Plane-parallel ion chamber	vented Plane-parallel ion chamber	Plane-parallel, liquid-filled ion chambers	liquid-filled ion chambers
Active Detector volume (mm^3)	5 × 5 × 3	4.4 × 4.4 × 3	2 × 2.5 × 2.5	2.3 × 2.3 × 0.5
Array Size (cm^2)	27 × 27	27 × 27	15 × 15	11 × 11
Detector Spacing center to center (mm)	10	7.1	2.5	2.5
Number of Detector	729	1405	1521	977
Repetition rate (ms)	100	100	100	100
Reference Point (mm)-Below the Surface Array	7.5	7.5	6.9	9
Array Geometry	Flat	Flat	Flat	Flat

Table 2.
List of ion chamber arrays manufactured by PTW dosimetry company [34].

The use of detector arrays reduces the amount of time required for physicists to perform pre-treatment verifications compared to using ion chamber- and film-based patient-specific QA. Many studies have examined various features of detector arrays and showed they are energy, dose rate, and angular independent plus serve as reliable dosimetry tools for pre-treatment verification of IMRT and VMAT [10, 35–39].

Detector arrays, however, have limited spatial resolutions, which can impact the accuracy of gamma passing rate results in small field dosimetry and detecting delivery errors. In 2018, Bruschi et al. [40] evaluated the effect of detector resolution on SBRT pre-treatment verification results. They compared three detectors (PTW OCTAVIUS 729, 1500, and 1000 SRS) in five different configurations with varying resolutions. These configurations included 729, merged 729, 1500, merged 1500, and 1000 SRS. The study evaluated 150 dose distributions in 30 plans, all of which were designed using Elekta Monaco® 5.0 TPS for a 10-MV X-ray beam on an Elekta Synergy® linac. The planned grid size was $2 \times 2 \times 2$ mm^3. Five types of error including systematic variations in collimator angle and gantry angle as well as lack of monitor units were introduced in order to establish the detection sensitivity of the three devices. This study demonstrated that the spatial resolution of the detector plays a vital role in SBRT QA. By increasing the spatial resolution of the detector, they reported that the average GPR value increases while reducing the spread of data. This happens due to small field dosimetry requiring high spatial resolution detectors. Moreover, the significance of detector spatial resolution was also dominant through an error detectability study. It was found that only the SRS array, with the highest resolution among the arrays used, was able to distinguish all the investigated errors [40]. Another study compared three detectors with different resolutions including ArcCHECK, MapCHECK2, and an electronic portal imaging device (EPID) to validate the dosimetric accuracy of the VMAT/IMRT QA [41]. First, they analyzed the performance of the three devices. Then, treatment plans from different treatment sites were assessed to evaluate the reliability of the detectors. Also, systematic variations such as MLC positioning were introduced to compare the detection sensitivity of the detectors. Then, the measurements were compared to the computed plan by TPS (Eclipse from Varian Medical Systems). The gamma analysis criteria of 3%/3, 2%/2, and 1%/1 mm with a dose threshold of 10% to remove the noise were used. Their findings indicated that both ArcCHECK and MapCHECK2 displayed the worst performance compared to EPID. This implies that low-spatial resolution can affect the gamma analysis due to under-sampling of the dose [41].

All these studies showed that the accuracy of the gamma passing rate depends on the detector resolution. Nevertheless, the gamma index method also has its sensitivity and limitations. Hence, it is crucial to carefully choose a detector with an appropriate resolution for the specific field size under investigation to prevent obtaining erroneous results.

2.2.4 Electronic portal imaging device

EPID was originally designed for visualization and patient setup in radiotherapy applications, but later on, it was discovered the digital image produced by EPID contains dose information that can be used for conducting routine QA of Linac and treatment verification. Its popularity and acceptance have been significantly bolstered by its high sensitivity, excellent spatial resolution, and the ability to instantly capture and present the delivered dose in digital format [42, 43]. In addition, analyzing the EPID image is much faster compared to film. The EPID is attached to the gantry of

Linac through a robotic arm so that it can intercept the exiting photon beam at all gantry angles to produce a digital image. The image can be acquired and displayed within seconds, which allows one to take multiple images during a treatment session. The EPID made of amorphous silicon (aSi) detector has been widely used among all available EPIDs due to faster image acquisition, high spatial resolution, high sensitivity, compact size, and stable response over time [43, 44]. Recently, Varian Medical Systems (Palo Alto, CA) has designed a new generation of digital megavolt imager called aS1200 EPID, which has a dosimetric active area of 40×40 cm^2 with 1280×1280-pixel arrays and a pixel size of 0.0336 cm. The device also includes extra backscatter shielding layers that minimize backscatter artifacts caused by the robotic support arm [43]. Removing the flattening filter from the beam path can increase the dose rate and central axis fluence, which can result in signal saturation [45]. Therefore, Varian Medical System has modified EPIDs for Flattening Filter Free (FFF) beams, ensuring no signal saturation occurs at any distance between the source and detector [42, 43]. This dosimetry system boasts the capability to measure dose rates up to 3200 MU/min, with an impressive acquisition rate of 25 frames per second. Furthermore, its analog-to-digital conversion bit is 16, rendering a separate digitization unit unnecessary for image preparation. Elekta company (Elekta AB, Stockholm, Sweden) has also developed the Elekta iViewGT panel, which is an aSi flat panel x-ray detector (XRD 1642 AP, Perkin Elmer Optoelectronics, Wiesbaden, Germany) and has an active imaging area of 41×41 cm^2 and a resolution of 1024×1024 16-bit pixels images with a pixel pitch of 400 μm and a nominal source to EPID distance of 160 cm [46].

Several studies have shown that EPID dosimetry is the most convenient tool for rapid and reliable patient-specific QA and can replace detector arrays in performing patient-specific QA of IMRT and VMAT, which can eliminate the need for phantom setup [47–54]. In 2019, Torres-Xirau et al. [55] investigated the dose response of EPID in the presence of a magnetic field using Unity MR-linac (Unity, Elekta AB, Stockholm, Sweden). The study concluded that the dose modeling of the EPID in the MR-Linac does not require any additional modifications due to the presence of a magnetic field. In other words, the presence of a magnetic field does not have a significant impact on the EPID responses [55].

2.3 Brachytherapy

Computed tomography or CT is usually used for dose calculation in modern brachytherapy. Although this technique has its merits, it is not enough to accurately assess the amount of radiation dose that reaches the tumor and surrounding organs during each treatment session. That is where *in-vivo* dosimetry (IVD) comes in and plays a crucial role in this field. *In-vivo* dosimetry is absorbed dose measurements in the patients while they are being treated. It helps to identify errors caused by equipment failure, dose calculation errors, applicator positioning errors, and changes in patient anatomy. In brachytherapy, IVD serves three purposes. Firstly, it aims to identify major deviations from the treatment plan that may impact the clinical outcome of the procedure. Secondly, it records minor deviations from the plan that cross a certain threshold, making it possible to modify the plan between treatments. Lastly, it also provides a reliable estimate of the actual delivered dose, which is invaluable for maintaining accurate patient records [56]. However, IVD in brachytherapy has several challenges such as high-dose gradients and appropriate positioning of the detector, the energy and dose rate dependence of the detector, and the possibility that an extra invasive procedure may be required. Therefore, the ideal detectors used for IVD should be small in volume to be placed close to the treated target to extract meaningful information and prevent dose averaging in high-dose gradient regions. Moreover, they should have a high signal-to-noise ratio, high spatial resolution, high dynamic range, energy and dose rate independence, reproducibility, linear dose-response over a broad range of energy, directional independence, real-time readouts, and wireless and affordability [57, 58]. The common detectors for clinical settings in brachytherapy are currently thermoluminescent dosimeters (TLDs), optically stimulated luminescence dosimeters (OSLD) (**Figure 2**), microDiamond, plastic Scintillation Detectors (PSDs), and semiconductor dosimeters (e.g., metal oxide semiconductor field effect transistors (MOSFETs)). Small-volume IC cannot be used since it does not have enough sensitivity to measure dose at centimeter distances from a ^{192}Ir source [59]. To measure the depth dependence, angular dependence, and temperature dependence of the detectors, a ^{192}Ir high dose-rate (HDR) brachytherapy source is usually used [57, 58].

Lithium fluoride (LiF), which is an alkali halide, is commonly used to construct TLDs. There are various physical forms of TLDs such as powder, cubical or cylindrical chips, rods, and pellets [60]. LiF TLD rods have been widely utilized for brachytherapy dosimetry due to easy insertion into catheters [58]. TLDs are the recommended detectors when measuring the AAPM TG-43 dosimetry parameters regarding low-energy photon-emitting brachytherapy sources. Because the validity of the absolute and relative dosimetry results of other detectors has not been persuasively demonstrated [57]. According to TG-43, $1 \times 1 \times 1$ cm^3 LiF TLD known as TLD 100 is a valid detector for absolute and relative dose measurements because its total combined uncertainty is low

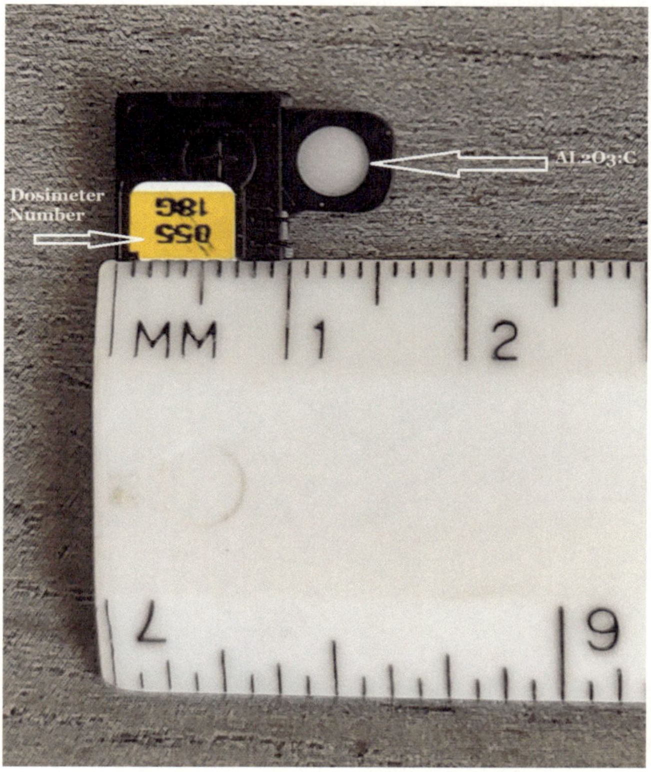

Figure 2.
Optically simulated luminescence dosimeters (OSLD).

(7 to 9 percent) [57]. TLD-100 chips are LiF crystals doped with titanium and magnesium in order to enhance the number of traps and luminescence centers [60]. TLDs are small, portable, have no bias needed to function, are affordable, cover a wide dose range, and have a small dose rate, energy, and temperature dependency [58]. However, there are some concerns associated with the use of TLDs, primarily the fact that they do not provide real-time measurements, which can lead to inaccuracies in dose measurements [59]. Also, they require a time-consuming preparation and readout process. In 2013, Horowitz and Moscovitch [61] showed that applying different readout parameters can impact the TLD response. Moreover, the positioning of TLD (LiF) for measurement [60, 62] and intrinsic energy dependence between ^{192}Ir and megavoltage calibration energy can be another source of uncertainty [62]. In recent years, OSLDs have been utilized more frequently as a potential alternative to TLDs. OSLDs are more affordable, smaller in size, and easier for patients' application than TLDs. OSLDs are usually placed in a plastic case ($10 \times 10 \times 2$ mm^3) infused with carbon-doped aluminum oxide (Al_2O_3:C). The detector is disk-shaped, 0.2 mm thick, and approximately 5 mm in diameter, with a mass density of 1.03 g/cm^3. The information is captured in an Al_2O_3:C and released by laser stimulation [63], which is much faster, more precise, and more reproducible compared to heating required for reading the TLDs [64]. The OSLD is optically bleached and can be reused multiple times until it reaches a cumulative dose of 10 Gy. The sensitivity decreases considerably once the radiation dose goes beyond 10 Gy [65]. The compact size of the OSLD makes it easy to fit into small and narrow spaces without visible volume-averaging effects.

Another detector that has gained popularity as an online in-vivo dosimeter is MOSFET. The Best® Medical Canada offers 3 different MOSFET dosimeters as standard MOSFET, microMOSFET, and Linear 5ive Array (**Figure 3**) with the active region of 0.2×0.2 mm and width of 2.5, 1, and 1.5 mm respectively. The linear five array is the recommended dosimeter for high-dose-rate and low-dose-rate

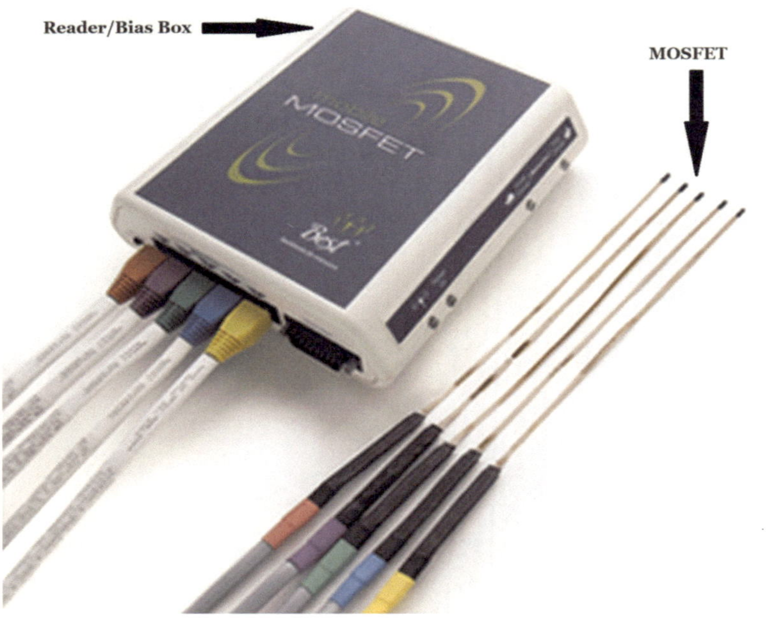

Figure 3.
MOSFET 5 Array. Best™ medical Canada [66]. (with permission).

brachytherapy by the manufacturer [66]. MOSFET is a semiconductor with three terminals: gate, drain, and source. They can be either n- or p-channel, but the p-channel MOSFETs are more common. In the p-channel, the source and drain are made of a p-type semiconductor and isolated from the gate by a layer of silicon dioxide (SiO_2). The gate is constructed using an n-type semiconductor. The sensitivity of a MOSFET detector's volume is determined by the SiO_2 insulator that captures electron-hole pairs during irradiation. The thickness of the silicon dioxide insulator can be varied between 0.1 to 1 μm, which affects the MOSFET's sensitivity [67]. Using a MOSFET dosimeter has several benefits, including its ability to accurately measure radiation doses in areas with steep dose gradients and cases of electronic disequilibrium due to its small detector size, lightweight design that poses no harm to patients, low power requirements, user-friendly operation, and real-time online readout [68–71]. The threshold voltage of its gate varies in proportion to the amount of absorption of radiation. The "threshold voltage" required for these devices is very low, and there is no risk of electrical shock [69]. The readings obtained from MOSFET indicate consistent results, displaying high dose linearity and insignificant fading [70, 71]. Zilio et al. [72] conducted a comparison between the dosimetry result of MOSFET and Monte Carlo calculations and confirmed the accuracy of the MOSFET dosimeter as an absolute dosimeter for brachytherapy. However, they are not water equivalent, have a limited lifetime, and do exhibit slight angular and depth dependence [69, 70]; therefore, care should be taken, and corrections must be applied for clinical applications.

Plastic Scintillation Detectors (PSDs) have also been used for IVD in brachytherapy [73, 74]. The PSDs are made up of plastic scintillating material with organic scintillating molecules dissolved in a polymerized solvent. This material emits light when exposed to ionizing radiation, and the amount of light produced is directly proportional to the radiation dose. The light is collected by optical fibers and converted into an electric charge that can be read by an electrometer [75]. In other words, the PSDs have four main components including a scintillating fiber that is a sensitive volume, a light pipe that is used to transmit scintillation photons, a photodetector, and an electrometer that is used for readout. PSDs have the advantage of being water equivalent, which makes them superior to inorganic detectors like MOSFETs or OSLDs [75, 76]. They are also flexible and waterproof and have high spatial resolution due to their small size, energy, angular independence, and dose linearity response [74–77]. Typically, PSDs are paired with photomultiplier tubes to provide real-time readouts [75].

MicroDiamond™ detector or mDD (e.g., Type 60,019 PTW-Freiburg, Germany) is another detector for IVD in brachytherapy that is a synthetic single-crystal diamond detector, with no bias voltage for operating [78]. This innovative synthetic diamond detector offers a perfect combination of the benefits found in natural diamond detectors and silicon diode detectors [79]. MicroDiamond detector is waterproof and has a spatial resolution of 4 mm^2, an active volume of 0.004 mm^3, and a thickness of 0.001 mm [79]. The effective point of measurement is 1mm away from its tip and has a nominal response of 1nC/Gy for Co-60. It exhibits a directional response in the water of less than $\pm$0.9% for radial incidence and less than $\pm$1% for axial incidence of $\pm$40°, making it a reliable tool for precise measurements [78]. The mDD was found to have the smallest energy-dependence among diodes and ICs [80]; much better water equivalence than p-type silicon diodes, ICs, and natural diamond detectors (PTW-60003-Freiburg, Germany) [78]; and also a lower absorbed-dose energy dependence compared to Si diodes and TLDs [81]. Moreover, the microDiamond detector displayed no dose-rate dependence effects observed in previous-generation natural diamond detectors [78].

It is worth noting that all detectors mentioned above are also utilized for external dosimetry of photon/electron and proton beams with energies falling within the radiotherapy range in external beam dosimetry.

2.4 Radiopharmaceutical

Radiopharmaceuticals are commonly used for both diagnostic imaging and radiation therapy. While they have the advantage of killing cancer cells, there are some levels of limitations to the use of these drugs due to damaging normal cells as well. Radiation dosages are optimized based on research studies performed on animals and clinical trials on human subjects before approval for clinical applications. Appropriate dosages are based on the careful study of pharmacokinetics, the physical characteristics of the radionuclide, the metabolism of the subject, and the pharmacodynamics of the radiopharmaceutical in animal and human subjects. The dosage is normally adjusted based on the weight of the patient or their total body surface area, with lower dosages recommended for children [82].

2.4.1 Radiopharmaceuticals approved by food and drug administration

Among the currently approved therapeutic radiopharmaceuticals by the Food and Drug Administration (FDA) commonly used ones' are Sodium iodide-131, Iobenguane iodine-131, Radium-223 dichloride, Yttrium-90 ibritumomab tiuxetan, Yttrium-90 microspheres, Strontium-89 chloride, Samarium-153 lexidronam, Lutetium-177 DOTATATE, and Lutetium-177 vipivotide tetraxetan [83].

Sodium iodine-131 has a half-life of approximately 8 days and decays by beta-particle emission (mean energy of 192 keV) to a stable ^{131}Xe. Sodium iodide-131 is used to treat thyroid carcinoma and hyperthyroidism (an overactive thyroid). It is available in liquid or capsule form and is absorbed mainly by the thyroid gland. The radiation from radioactive iodine damages the thyroid gland, reducing its activity to normal levels. Radioiodide is used in larger doses after thyroid cancer surgery to destroy any remaining diseased thyroid tissue or to destroy thyroid cancer that has spread to other tissues. Small doses of radioactivity help physicians to determine whether the thyroid gland is working properly or locate tumors caused by certain types of thyroid cancers [84].

Iobenguane-iodine-131 or AZERDA® (Progenics Pharmaceuticals) is a radioactive agent used for the treatment of pheochromocytoma or paraganglioma. Adults and children older than 12 years old with iobenguane scan positive, unresectable, locally advanced or metastatic pheochromocytoma or paraganglioma who require systemic anticancer therapy are common candidates for iobenguane iodine-131 therapy [85].

Radium-223 dichloride, sold under the brand name Xofigo® (Bayer), is used to treat prostate cancer that has spread only to the bony anatomy and is symptomatic and no longer responds to hormonal or surgical treatment that lowers testosterone. Radium-223 dichloride is primarily an alpha particle emitter with a half-life of 11.4 days. The energy range of alpha particles emitted from Ra-223 and its daughter is from 5.0 to 7.7 MeV [86].

Yttrium ibritumomab tiuxetan (^{90}Y-IT) or ZEVAKIN® contains a radioactive substance called Yttrium-90 (^{90}Y) to treat certain types of B-cell non-Hodgkin lymphoma (NHL) or previously untreated follicular NHL who get a partial or complete response to first-line chemotherapy. Yttrium-90 emits beta particles (2.28 MeV) with a physical half-life of 64.1 hours (2.67 days) [83, 87].

Yttrium-90 microspheres are radioactive particles employed for treating patients with unresectable hepatocellular carcinoma (HCC) or liver cancer. In the United States, the Yttrium-90 Microspheres that are commercially available are TheraSphere® (glass microspheres, Boston Scientific Corporation), and SIR-Spheres® (resin microspheres, Sirtex Medical Ltd) [83].

Samarium-153 lexidronam contains samarium-153, which emits medium-energy beta particles and an imageable gamma photon with a physical half-life of 46.3 hours and maximum energy of 0.808 MeV. Radioactive samarium is used to alleviate bone pain in certain types of cancer by emitting radiation in the affected area.

Strontium-89 chloride (the common name of Metastron) is a radioisotope agent that may be used to diagnose some diseases by studying the function of the body's organs or be used to treat certain diseases. When used in therapy, it is injected into patients intravenously to deliver radiation to cancer sites and ultimately decreases bone pain. The radioactive strontium is taken up in the bone cancer area and gives off radiation that helps provide relief of pain. Metastron decays by beta emission with a physical half-life of 50.5 days. The maximum beta energy is 1.463 MeV (100%). The maximum range of β- from Strontium-89 in tissue is approximately 8 mm.

Lutetium Lu 177 dotatate (LUTATHERA, Advanced Accelerator Applications USA, Inc.) contains LU-177, which has a physical half-life of 6.647 days and emits beta particles with maximum energy of 0.498 MeV and average energy of 0.133 MeV and gamma rays [88]. Lutetium Lu 177 dotatate is a radiopharmaceutical used to treat adult patients with either metastatic or inoperable cancer known as gastroenteropancreatic neuroendocrine tumors (GEP-NETs) that are positive for the hormone receptor somatostatin, including GEP-NETs in the foregut, midgut, and hindgut [83].

Lutetium-177 (177Lu) Vipivotide Tetraxetan (PLUVICTO®, Novartis/Advanced Accelerator Applications) is a radioconjugate composed of prostate-specific membrane antigen (PSMA)-targeting ligand, combined with Lu-177, a beta-emitting radioisotope, to potentially combat tumor cells that express PSMA.

All radiopharmaceuticals should only be administered by authorized personnel in designated clinical settings after patient evaluation by a qualified physician.

2.4.2 Internal radiation dosimetry

The field of internal radiation dosimetry focuses on measuring the amount of radiation energy deposited in the body's tissue by radionuclides. This involves examining the physical characteristics of radionuclides, as well as their pharmacokinetics and biokinetics [82]. One of the standard techniques to assess internal radiation doses from the administered radiopharmaceuticals in target organs is known as medical internal radiation dosimetry or MIRD. The MIRD system for calculating doses follows a structured method that utilizes information on the biological distribution of radiopharmaceuticals, the clearance rate of radiopharmaceuticals from the body, and the physical characteristics of radionuclides [82]. This approach is based on the absorbed dose method and provides more accurate results compared to other techniques. The MIRD method uses a simple model of the human body and includes source organs and target organs. The "target organ" is the recipient of the radiated energy from the source organs, and the "source organ" is any organ other than the target organ that contains radiopharmaceuticals. An organ can be both a target and a source [89]. In this case, the energy deposited in that organ is called self-dose.

The absorbed dose is calculated based on Eq. (14).

$$Absorbed\ Dose = \frac{Energy\ Absorbed\ from\ Ionizing\ Radiation}{Mass\ of\ Organ} \tag{14}$$

The unit of absorbed dose in the international system of Units (SI) is "*gray*" or "*Gy*," which is equal to 1-joule energy absorbed per 1 Kg of absorber material. Its traditional unit is "*rad*" and is used more commonly in the United States. 1 rad is 100 ergs of energy absorbed per gram of medium; therefore, 1 rad = 0.01 Gy.

The amount of absorbed dose is influenced by various factors. These factors consist of the quantity of radioactivity present in the source organ, the duration for which radioactivity resides in the source organ, the type and quantity of radiation energy released by radioactivity in the source organ, and the proportion of the energy emitted by the source that is absorbed by the target organ.

To calculate the absorbed dose using the MIRD method, we need to quantify each abovementioned component step by step.

Step 1. Cumulated Activity, Ã

The amount of radiation received by a target organ depends on the level of radioactivity in the source organ and the time length that the radioactivity resides in the source organ. The product of these two factors is the cumulated activity (Ã) in the source organ, which can be written as Eq. 15 and has a unit of μCi-hr.

$$\tilde{A} = \int_0^\infty A(t)dt \tag{15}$$

Where A(t) is the radioactivity in a source organ over time of t (**Figure 4**). A(t) is different from person to person and varies in each organ. However, in human studies, it can be estimated through various methods, such as animal studies, which are then extrapolated with some uncertainty to humans. Additionally, imaging studies in normal human subjects and prior knowledge of the tracer kinetics are also utilized, sometimes in combination, to obtain these estimates [90]. A simplified mathematical model for A(t) can be described as:

$$A(t) = A_0 e^{-\lambda_e t} \tag{16}$$

where $\lambda_e = \lambda_p + \lambda_b$.

λ_e, λ_p, and λ_b are the effective, physical decay, and biologic decay constants, respectively.

The decay constant can be calculated based on the half-life using Eq. 17.

$$\lambda = \frac{0.693}{T_{1/2}} \tag{17}$$

Therefore, cumulated activity is equal to

$$\tilde{A} = \frac{A_0}{\lambda_e} = 1.44 T_e A_0 \tag{18}$$

where T_e is the effective half-life and A_0 is the initial administered activity.

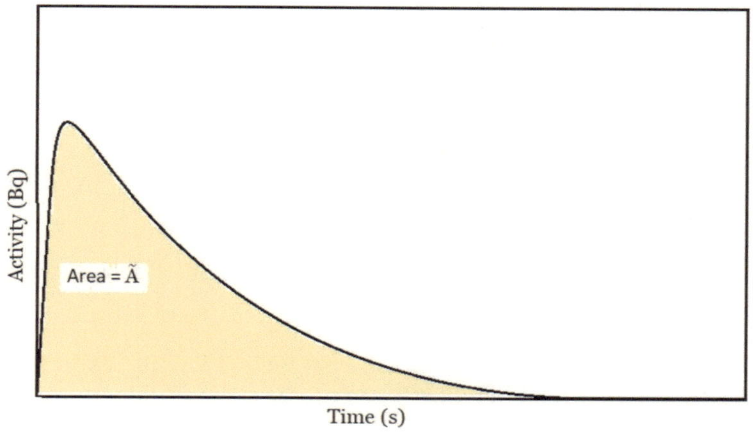

Figure 4.
A hypothetical time-activity curve that shows the level of radioactivity in a specific organ over time.

Step 2. Equilibrium Absorbed Dose Constant, Δ

After calculating the value of Ã, the next step is to determine the amount of radiation energy emitted by this cumulated activity. The amount of energy emitted per unit of cumulated activity in the source organ is given by the equilibrium absorbed dose constant Δ. This factor must be determined for each type of emission for the radionuclide and can be calculated using Eq. 19.

$$\Delta_i = kN_iE_i \tag{19}$$

where E_i is the average energy of the emission i^{th}, expressed in the unit of MeV, and N_i is the relative frequency of that emission. The value of k in the SI unit is 1.6×10^{-13} and in the traditional unit is 2.13. The units for Δ is Gy.kg/Bq.sec. and rad. g/μCi.hr. in SI and traditional units, respectively. Therefore, the radiation energy emitted by the source activity cumulated over time is given by $\tilde{A} \times \Delta$.

Step 3. Absorbed Fraction, ϕ

The energy absorbed by a target (r_k) from a source region (r_h) irradiation is:

$$\tilde{A} \times \Delta_i \times \Phi_i \tag{20}$$

Where ϕ represents the absorbed fraction, which indicates the proportion of energy released by the source and deposited in the target. The amount of radiation energy that reaches the target organ depends on its composition (e.g., lung, bone) and volume, as well as the distance attenuation between the source and target organs. This means that the absorbed fraction is influenced by the type and energy of the emission, as well as the anatomical relationship between the source and target pair. When performing a dosimetry calculation, it is necessary to determine a value of ϕ for each type of emission from the radionuclide and each source-target pair in the calculation.

The total energy absorbed can be mathematically expressed as:

$$\tilde{A} \sum_i \phi_i (r_k \leftarrow r_h) \Delta_i \tag{21}$$

The notation ϕ_i ($r_k \leftarrow r_h$) represents the absorbed fraction of energy delivered to the target organ (r_k) from a source organ or region (r_h) for the ith emission of the radionuclide.

Now, the absorbed dose equation can be written as follows:

$$D(r_k \leftarrow r_h) = \frac{\tilde{A}}{mass\ of\ the\ target\ (m_k)} \sum_i \phi_i (r_k \leftarrow r_h) \Delta_i \tag{22}$$

The total dose of the target organ then is the summation of doses from all source organs inside the body.

Step 4. S-Factor

The S-factor is a measure of radiation dose per unit of activity, expressed in Gy/Bq. sec. The S-factor can be found in tables based on the radionuclide, source organ, and target organ. The MIRD pamphlet No.11 [91] tabulated many of the most used radionuclides for the standard phantom (The MIRD phantom is a simplified model of a 70 kg adult male) and expressed them in the conventional unit of rad/μCi.hr. Eq. 22 can be divided into two parts: (a) cumulated activity (Ã) and (b) factors that depend on radionuclide properties and the size and position of different organs in the phantom model. This latter quantity is called the S factor, and it is defined mathematically.

$$S(r_k \leftarrow r_h) = \frac{\sum_i \phi_i (r_k \leftarrow r_h) \Delta_i}{m_k} \tag{23}$$

If we define a specific absorbed fraction as follows:

$$\Phi = \frac{\phi_i}{m_k} \tag{24}$$

then dose equation can be simplified as:

$$\overline{D}(r_k \leftarrow r_h) = \tilde{A} \times S(r_k \leftarrow r_h) \tag{25}$$

where S is S-factor, or the mean absorbed dose per cumulated activity.

Step 5. Effective Dose Calculation

The effective dose to the whole body is given by Eq. (26).

$$E = \sum_T W_T D_T W_R = \sum_T W_T H_T \tag{26}$$

The unit used for measuring the effective dose, E, is Sievert. D_T and W_T are the average absorbed dose and tissue equivalent factor for organ T. W_R is equal to unity for all radiations used in diagnostic nuclear medicine such as gamma rays, X-rays, electrons, and positrons. The equivalent dose, H_T, specifies a quantity that considers the relative biologic damage caused by radiation with a particular tissue or organ and is given by Eq. (27).

$$H_T = D_T W_R \tag{27}$$

The unit of H_T is also Sievert, so care must be taken to use this unit as it is associated with both equivalent dose and effective dose. The effective dose is primarily designed for assessing radiation risks and measuring radiation doses received by workers in the radiation industry. It can also be applied to clinical nuclear medicine. The effective dose demonstrates the total body dose that would cause the same overall risk as the nonuniform dose distribution delivered. This is accomplished by assigning different weighting factors to the doses received by individual organs [89].

3. Proton therapy dosimetry

The primary distinction between photon and proton beams lies in the inherent physical characteristics of the proton beam. Protons are directly ionizing charged particles with a positive charge and a finite range. Consequently, proton and photon beams have a completely different dose distribution. Unlike photons, protons release an immense amount of energy at the end of their path and produce a maximum peak near the end of their range. The maximum peak is called the "Bragg peak," which is a distinct property of protons, and the proton dose falls to zero instantly beyond the Bragg peak. This can be used to increase the dose to targets while minimizing radiation exposure to normal tissue [92, 93]. Correspondingly, it is a crucial task to determine the location of the dose deposition to ensure the target, not OARs, received the prescribed dose. This information can be extracted using IVD. In both brachytherapy and proton therapy, various detectors play a crucial role in ensuring accurate and safe treatment delivery. These detectors include MOSFET (Metal-Oxide-Semiconductor Field-Effect Transistor), PSD (Position-Sensitive Detector), OSLD (Optically Stimulated Luminescence Dosimeter), TLD (Thermoluminescent Dosimeter), and microDiamond. MOSFET detectors are valued for their real-time response and sensitivity, making them suitable for measuring dose distribution during treatment. PSDs are used to determine the position of charged particles in the proton beam, contributing to beam monitoring and verification. OSLDs and TLDs, as passive detectors, are employed to measure the absorbed dose of ionizing radiation in both modalities. MicroDiamond detectors, with their high spatial resolution, offer valuable insights into dose delivery and beam characteristics in proton therapy. While the applications of these detectors are similar in both brachytherapy and proton therapy, their specific utilization may vary depending on the treatment facility's protocols and equipment. Up-to-date research and consultation with experts in the field are essential to stay informed about the latest advancements and best practices [94–98]. However, these approaches are only applicable when the detectors could be placed on the skin or accessible body cavities (e.g., in prostate cancer where dosimeters can be located inside the rectum).

The dose or range of proton can also be monitored using imaging methods such as positron emission tomography (PET), prompt gamma (PG) imaging, ionoacoustic imaging, and follow-up MRI. Due to the lack of exit dose in proton therapy, EPID cannot be used.

The in-vivo range verification with PET can be performed online (in-beam) monitoring or offline. In the online technique, a small field-of-view dual head PET is attached to the gantry, allowing taking images during or immediately after treatment, while in the offline method, the patient is transferred to the PET/CT scanner room after treatment. The reason for using PET is that protons collide with atoms in tissues (non-elastic collision), causing nuclear reactions that create positrons ($^{+}\beta$). Combining the information from the PET image with the patient's anatomy can provide data to determine the location of the positron emitters in the patient's body to identify the path of the proton beam and monitor the location of the tumor and dose deposition path [99–101].

Prompt gamma imaging is the second approach for providing real-time in-vivo range verification of the proton using a Compton camera [102–106]. The camera detects MeV prompt γ-rays emitted from excited nuclei along the proton path to create an image using two stages of detectors. The first stage includes photon-scattering detectors, while the second stage has photon-absorbing detectors [105]. Data obtained from the energy deposition and spatial coordinates of gamma rays, resulting from at least two interactions in the stages of Charged-Particle Cancer Therapy (CC), could potentially be utilized to precisely determine the range of the ion beam with an accuracy of up to 1 millimeter. In this context, Charged-Particle Cancer Therapy refers to a treatment modality that employs charged particles, such as protons or heavy ions, to target cancer cells with high precision and minimal damage to surrounding healthy tissues. When these charged particles interact with the patient's tissue, they produce secondary particles, including gamma rays, through nuclear interactions. By carefully analyzing the energy and spatial information of these gamma rays from multiple interactions, medical physicists and radiation therapists can gain valuable insights into the distribution of the ion beam within the patient's body. This data can be processed using advanced algorithms and computational techniques to accurately determine the range of the charged particles, helping to ensure that the tumor receives the prescribed radiation dose while sparing nearby healthy tissues. This level of accuracy in determining the ion beam range is of utmost importance in radiation therapy to maximize the treatment's effectiveness and minimize potential side effects. It allows for precise treatment planning and delivery, leading to better outcomes for cancer patients undergoing Charged-Particle Cancer Therapy [104, 107].

A third technique for range verification in proton therapy is ionoacoustic, a non-nuclear technique [107–109]. This approach is a direct technique to localize the Bragg peak based on the thermoacoustic effect. The local energy deposition of a pulsed ion beam within a short time (μsec) in a limited tissue volume (mm^3) can generate an ultrasound signal (ionoacoustic signal) with a frequency in the of range 0.1 to 10 MHz. Detecting this signal allows the user to precisely localize the Bragg peak's position [107, 108].

The fourth approach is to use MRI under certain conditions to determine in-vivo range verification of proton [110–113]. One well-known example is the use of MRI to detect the fatty conversion in the vertebral bone marrow after proton therapy to visualize the proton beam and its range [111]. A similar observation has also been reported for changes in the liver [110]. This technique is a late approach, usually 3 to 6 months after proton therapy [110].

In summary, these imaging techniques for in-vivo range verification in proton therapy look promising, but they are still in the research and developmental phase.

4. Neutron therapy dosimetry

Neutrons can penetrate tissues deeply and can interact with atomic nuclei, releasing energy that damages cancer cells and have a higher relative biological effectiveness (RBE) compared to photons. This means that neutron radiation can cause more significant damage to cancer cells per unit of absorbed dose, potentially improving treatment outcomes.

The three different techniques for neutron therapy in radiation oncology are: (a) ^{252}Cf neutron brachytherapy, (b) Fast neutron therapy (FNT), and (c) Boron neutron capture therapy (BNCT).

4.1 ^{252}Cf neutron brachytherapy

The isotope Californium-252 is a source of gamma/neutron radiation with a half-life of 2.645 years and was introduced for brachytherapy in the late 1960s and early 1970s [114]. This form of brachytherapy is particularly useful for treating deep-seated tumors that are challenging to reach with other radiation sources. ^{252}Cf was usually used in combination with external photon beam therapy since it was discovered that irradiating tumors with ^{252}Cf before photon irradiation is more effective [115]. Currently, ^{252}Cf is not being clinically implanted due to its large size and low activity levels [114].

4.2 Fast neutron therapy

Fast neutron therapy was common during the 1980s and 1990s and became an available option to treat certain tumors such as advanced prostate cancer [116], breast cancer [117], and bone and soft tissue sarcomas [118–120]. Fast neutrons are the production of one of the nuclear reactions such as fusion interaction (d + T or d + D), stripping reactions (d + Be), and inelastic interactions (p + Be). Among all these nuclear reactions, p + Be is the most preferable option for modern, high-energy facilities [121].

4.3 Boron neutron capture therapy

Boron neutron capture therapy (BNCT) is a radiotherapy technique to eradicate tumors such as melanoma, brain tumors, and head and neck cancers. This treatment is based on the nuclear reaction known as boron neutron capture ($^{10}B\ (n, \alpha)^{7}Li$) in which boron-10 absorbs low thermal neutrons (<0.5 eV), resulting in the production of helium nuclei ($^{4}He_2$) and recoiling lithium-7 ($^{7}Li_3$) atoms [122, 123]. These particles deposit energy in a short range (<10 μm) due to the high linear energy transfer, which results in substantial damage to malignant cells accumulated with boron-10 [124].

4.4 Neutron therapy dosimetry

Neutron fields are usually a mixture of photon and neutron, which makes the dosimetry more complicated. Neutrons like photons ionize indirectly; however, they have different RBE; hence, it is necessary to measure them separately [125, 126]. In neutron dosimetry, the energy of the neutron and the composition of the tissue (hydrogen, carbon, nitrogen, oxygen, calcium, and phosphorus) for dosimetry are key factors. Because the probability of interaction between the neutron and the element within the body depends on the neutron energy and the target nuclide. Neutrons are classified based on their energies nevertheless; there is no agreement to classify them precisely. The following is an approximation:

- Thermal (0.025 eV)
- Slow (<10 eV)

- Intermediate (10 eV – 100 keV)
- Fast (>100 keV)

The recommended dosimetry method to measure the absorbed dose in fast-neutron fields is described by the international commission on radiation units and Measurements (ICRU) protocol No. 45 using an ion chamber [127]. The tissue equivalent material should be used for the wall, gas, electrode, and water for the phantom. The absorbed dose is computed based on the application of the Bragg-Gray cavity theory (Eq. 28).

$$D = \frac{Q_n}{m} \times \frac{W_n}{e} \left(r_{m,g}\right)_n d_T \frac{1}{1+\delta} \tag{28}$$

Where Q is the charge of one sign produced in the cavity, and W_n is the average amount of energy required to form an ion pair. This value is calculated as a mean for all the charged particles that are produced during neutron interactions in the gas material being used. $(r_{m,g})_n$ is the gas-to-wall absorbed-dose conversion factor; d_T is the displacement correction factor, and δ is a correction factor to account for the difference in the response of the detector, such as the ionization chamber, to different types of radiation, such as neutrons and photons [127]. Another detector is a low-pressure Tissue Equivalent Proportional Counter (TEPC), which can be used for BNCT measurements and is able to measure the absorbed dose and information about the microscopic nature and beam quality [128]. However, collecting data with TEPC is slow and time-consuming. To obtain beam data more efficiently, a set of three ion chambers including an A-150 TEP chamber, an Mg chamber, and another Mg chamber filled with B-10 on its inner surface were usually utilized [128]. The Si diodes can also be used for neutron dosimetry since their sensitivity to photons is negligible. They also have higher spatial resolution compared to ion chambers, which can improve penumbra measurements [125, 129]. Another method used for in-vivo dosimetry of neutrons includes the use of activation detectors. These detectors contain materials that activate when exposed to neutrons, resulting in the emission of gamma rays. The intensity of the gamma rays can be measured, indicating the neutron dose. TLDs and solid-state detectors can also be used for in-vivo neutron dosimetry.

Unfortunately, due to advanced development in photon and proton therapy, neutron therapy is not a common cancer therapy technique at the time of this writing. Therefore, obtaining updated information about the dosimetry of this treatment technique is quite challenging.

5. Conclusion

In this chapter of the book, we have presented a concise outline of sophisticated methodologies and tools employed in the field of dosimetry, primarily emphasizing the assessment of photon and electron dosages. Distinctive detectors exhibit variations in their performance across diverse dosimetric situations, encompassing factors like small versus large fields, low versus high spatial detector precision, or the use of photon versus proton beams. The utilization of an inappropriate detector could result in inaccurate quality assurance outcomes. Consequently, it is imperative for medical physicists to possess a comprehensive understanding of detector constraints when quantifying doses, thereby ensuring precision in clinical applications.

DOI: http://dx.doi.org/10.5772/intechopen.1002727

Author details

Elahheh Salari[1] and E. Ishmael Parsai[2*]

1 Emory University School of Medicine, Atlanta, Georgia, USA

2 University of Toledo Medical Center, Toledo, Ohio, USA

*Address all correspondence to: ishmael.parsai@gmail.com

References

[1] Almond PR, Biggs PJ, Coursey BM, Hanson WF, Huq MS, Nath R, et al. AAPM's TG-51 protocol for clinical reference dosimetry of high-energy photon and electron beams. Medical Physics. 1999;**26**(9):1847-1870

[2] McEwen M, DeWerd L, Ibbott G, Followill D, Rogers DW, Seltzer S, et al. Addendum to the AAPM's TG-51 protocol for clinical reference dosimetry of high-energy photon beams. Medical Physics. 2014;**41**(4):041501

[3] Knoll GF. Radiation Detection and Measurement. 4th ed. John Wiley & Sons, Inc.; 2010. 864 p

[4] Mettler FA, Guiberteau MJ. 2 - instrumentation and quality control. In: Mettler FA, Guiberteau MJ, editors. Essentials of Nuclear Medicine and Molecular Imaging. Seventh ed. Philadelphia: Elsevier; 2019. pp. 19-59

[5] Palmans H, Andreo P, Huq MS, Seuntjens J, Christaki KE, Meghzifene A. Dosimetry of small static fields used in external photon beam radiotherapy: Summary of TRS-483, the IAEA–AAPM international code of practice for reference and relative dose determination. Medical Physics. 2018; **45**(11):e1123-e1145

[6] Fraser D, Parker W, Seuntjens J. Characterization of cylindrical ionization chambers for patient specific IMRT QA. Journal of Applied Clinical Medical Physics. 2009;**10**(4):241-251

[7] Salari E, Shuai XK, Sperling NN, Parsai EI. Using machine learning to predict gamma passing rate in volumetric-modulated arc therapy treatment plans. Journal of Applied Clinical Medical Physics. 2023;**24**(2): e13824

[8] Xu Y, Zhang K, Liu Z, Liang B, Ma X, Ren W, et al. Treatment plan prescreening for patient-specific quality assurance measurements using independent Monte Carlo dose calculations. Frontiers in Oncology. 2022;**12**:1051110

[9] Leybovich LB, Sethi A, Dogan N. Comparison of ionization chambers of various volumes for IMRT absolute dose verification. Medical Physics. 2003; **30**(2):119-123

[10] Parsai EI, Salari E. Ch. 3. Parameters affecting pre-treatment dosimetry verification. In: Thomas JF, Maryann B-J, editors. Dosimetry. Rijeka: IntechOpen; 2022

[11] Fenoglietto P, Laliberté B, Aillères N, Riou O, Dubois J-B, Azria D. Eight years of IMRT quality assurance with ionization chambers and film dosimetry: Experience of the Montpellier comprehensive cancer center. Radiation Oncology. 2011;**6**(1):85

[12] Syam Kumar SA, Sukumar P, Sriram P, Rajasekaran D, Aketi S, Vivekanandan N. A patient-specific quality assurance study on absolute dose verification using ionization chambers of different volumes in RapidArc treatments. Medical Dosimetry. 2012; **37**(4):436-441

[13] Ocadiz A, Livingstone J, Donzelli M, Bartzsch S, Nemoz C, Kefs S, et al. Film dosimetry studies for patient specific quality assurance in microbeam radiation therapy. Physica Medica. 2019; **65**:227-237

[14] Wen N, Lu S, Kim J, Qin Y, Huang Y, Zhao B, et al. Precise film dosimetry for stereotactic radiosurgery and stereotactic body radiotherapy

quality assurance using Gafchromic EBT3 films. Radiation Oncology. 2016; **11**(1):132

[15] Reinhardt S, Hillbrand M, Wilkens JJ, Assmann W. Comparison of Gafchromic EBT2 and EBT3 films for clinical photon and proton beams. Medical Physics. 2012;**39**(8):5257-5262

[16] Casanova Borca V, Pasquino M, Russo G, Grosso P, Cante D, Sciacero P, et al. Dosimetric characterization and use of GAFCHROMIC EBT3 film for IMRT dose verification. Journal of Applied Clinical Medical Physics. 2013; **14**(2):4111

[17] Ashland, KY. Gafchromic radiotherapy films: Available from: http://www.ashland.com/products/gafchromic-radiotherapy-films.

[18] Buchauer K, Hillbrand E, de Vries A. GAFCHROMIC EBT photospectral dose response dependence on temperature and implications for flat bed scanning. Medical Physics. 2009;**36**(11):5044-5051

[19] Villarreal-Barajas JE, Khan RF. Energy response of EBT3 radiochromic films: Implications for dosimetry in kilovoltage range. Journal of Applied Clinical Medical Physics. 2014;**15**(1): 4439

[20] Bassi S, Cummins D, McCavana P. Energy and dose dependence of GafChromic EBT3-V3 film across a wide energy range. Reports of Practical Oncology & Radiotherapy. 2020;**25**(1): 60-63

[21] Sipilä P, Ojala J, Kaijaluoto S, Jokelainen I, Kosunen A. Gafchromic EBT3 film dosimetry in electron beams - energy dependence and improved film read-out. Journal of Applied Clinical Medical Physics. 2016; **17**(1):360-373

[22] Ataei G, Rezaei M, Gorji KE, Banaei A, Goushbolagh NA, Farhood B, et al. Evaluation of dose rate and photon energy dependence of Gafchromic EBT3 film irradiating with 6 MV and Co-60 photon beams. Journal of Medical Signals and Sensors. 2019;**9**(3):204-210

[23] Gungor G, Korkmaz L, Kayalilar N Sr, Aydin G, Yapici B, Zoto Mustafayev T, et al. Multichannel film dosimetry for quality assurance of intensity modulated radiotherapy treatment plans under 0.35 T magnetic field. Cureus. 2020;**12**(3):e7334

[24] Low DA, Dempsey JF. Evaluation of the gamma dose distribution comparison method. Medical Physics. 2003;**30**(9): 2455-2464

[25] James S, Al-Basheer A, Elder E, Huh C, Ackerman C, Barrett J, et al. Evaluation of commercial devices for patient specific QA of stereotactic radiotherapy plans. Journal of Applied Clinical Medical Physics. 2023;**24**(8): e14009

[26] Miura H, Ozawa S, Hosono F, Sumida N, Okazue T, Yamada K, et al. Gafchromic EBT-XD film: Dosimetry characterization in high-dose, volumetric-modulated arc therapy. Journal of Applied Clinical Medical Physics. 2016;**17**(6):312-322

[27] Grams MP, Gustafson JM, Long KM, de Los Santos LE. Technical note: Initial characterization of the new EBT-XD Gafchromic film. Medical Physics. 2015; **42**(10):5782-5786

[28] Devic S. Radiochromic film dosimetry: Past, present, and future. Physica Medica. 2011;**27**(3):122-134

[29] Devic S, Tomic N, Aldelaijan S, DeBlois F, Seuntjens J, Chan MF, et al. Linearization of dose–response curve of

the radiochromic film dosimetry system. Medical Physics. 2012;**39**(8):4850-4857

[30] Devic S, Tomic N, Lewis D. Reference radiochromic film dosimetry: Review of technical aspects. Physica Medica. 2016;**32**(4):541-556

[31] Mathot M, Sobczak S, Hoornaert MT. Gafchromic film dosimetry: Four years experience using FilmQA pro software and Epson flatbed scanners. Physica Medica. 2014;**30**(8): 871-877

[32] Russo S, Masi L, Francescon P, Frassanito MC, Fumagalli ML, Marinelli M, et al. Multicenter evaluation of a synthetic single-crystal diamond detector for CyberKnife small field size output factors. Physica Medica. 2016; **32**(4):575-581

[33] Pre-treatment Delivery: SUN NUCLEAR Corporation. Available from: https://www.sunnuclear.com/products.

[34] OCTAVIUS Phantom: PTW, The Dosimetry Company. Available from: https://www.ptwdosimetry.com/en/products/octavius-4d-qa-phantom.

[35] Li JG, Yan G, Liu C. Comparison of two commercial detector arrays for IMRT quality assurance. Journal of Applied Clinical Medical Physics. 2009; **10**(2):62-74

[36] Popple RA, Sullivan RJ, Yuan Y, Wu X, Covington EL. Evaluation of a two-dimensional diode array for patient-specific quality assurance of HyperArc. Journal of Applied Clinical Medical Physics. 2021;**22**(12):203-210

[37] Salari E, Parsai EI, Shvydka D, Sperling NN. Evaluation of parameters affecting gamma passing rate in patient-specific QAs for multiple brain lesions IMRS treatments using ray-station treatment planning system. Journal of Applied Clinical Medical Physics. 2022; **23**(1):e13467

[38] Aristophanous M, Suh Y, Chi PC, Whittlesey LJ, LaNeave S, Martel MK. Initial clinical experience with ArcCHECK for IMRT/VMAT QA. Journal of Applied Clinical Medical Physics. 2016;**17**(5):20-33

[39] Thiyagarajan R, Nambiraj A, Sinha SN, Yadav G, Kumar A, Subramani V, et al. Analyzing the performance of ArcCHECK diode array detector for VMAT plan. Reports of Practical Oncology & Radiotherapy. 2016;**21**(1):50-56

[40] Bruschi A, Esposito M, Pini S, Ghirelli A, Zatelli G, Russo S. How the detector resolution affects the clinical significance of SBRT pre-treatment quality assurance results. Physica Medica. 2018;**49**:129-134

[41] Woon W, Ravindran PB, Ekayanake PSV, Lim YY, Khalid J. A study on the effect of detector resolution on gamma index passing rate for VMAT and IMRT QA. Journal of Applied Clinical Medical Physics. 2018;**19**(2): 230-248

[42] Miri N, Keller P, Zwan BJ, Greer P. EPID-based dosimetry to verify IMRT planar dose distribution for the aS1200 EPID and FFF beams. Journal of Applied Clinical Medical Physics. 2016;**17**(6): 292-304

[43] Subramani V, Rathakrishnan M, Nambiraj NA, Chitra S, Venkatraman M. Dosimetric validation of digital megavolt imager for flattening filter free beams in the pre-treatment quality assurance of stereotactic body radiation therapy for liver metastases. Asian Pacific Journal of Cancer Prevention. 2020;**21**(6): 1659-1665

[44] Ma Y, Wang X, Mai R, Wang T, Pei Y, Liu S, et al. An electronic portal image device (EPID)-based multiplatform rapid daily LINAC QA tool. Journal of Applied Clinical Medical Physics. 2021;**22**(1):45-58

[45] Parsai EI, Pearson D, Kvale T. Consequences of removing the flattening filter from linear accelerators in generating high dose rate photon beams for clinical applications: A Monte Carlo study verified by measurement. Nuclear Instruments and Methods in Physics Research Section B: Beam Interactions with Materials and Atoms. 2007;**261**(1): 755-759

[46] Elekta. Save time and increase confidence with Elekta Patient QA Solutions. Available from: https://www.elekta.com/

[47] Alharthi T, Vial P, Holloway L, Thwaites D. Intrinsic detector sensitivity analysis as a tool to characterize ArcCHECK and EPID sensitivity to variations in delivery for lung SBRT VMAT plans. Journal of Applied Clinical Medical Physics. 2021;**22**(6):229-240

[48] Bidaut LM, Humm JL, Mageras GS. Rothenberg LN. 8 - imaging in radiation oncology, This chapter is an update and expansion of material presented in the first edition by Ling CC, Mohan R, Reinstein LE, Rothenberg LN. In: Hoppe RT, Phillips TL, Roach M, editors. Leibel and Phillips Textbook of Radiation Oncology. Third ed. Philadelphia: W.B. Saunders; 2010. pp. 120-154 and in the second edition by the current authors

[49] Grządziel A, Smolińska B, Rutkowski R, Ślosarek K. EPID dosimetry – Configuration and pre-treatment IMRT verification. Reports of Practical Oncology & Radiotherapy. 2007;**12**(6):307-312

[50] Miri N, Legge K, Colyvas K, Lehmann J, Vial P, Moore A, et al. A remote EPID-based dosimetric TPS-planned audit of centers for clinical trials: Outcomes and analysis of contributing factors. Radiation Oncology. 2018;**13**(1):178

[51] Nailon WH, Welsh D, McDonald K, Burns D, Forsyth J, Cooke G, et al. EPID-based in vivo dosimetry using dosimetry check™: Overview and clinical experience in a 5-yr study including breast, lung, prostate, and head and neck cancer patients. Journal of Applied Clinical Medical Physics. 2019;**20**(1):6-16

[52] Nasseri S, Bahreyni MH, Momennezhad M, Gholamhosseinian H, Shahedi F, Hashemi SM, et al. Dosimetric verification of IMRT and 3D conformal treatment delivery using EPID. Applied Radiation and Isotopes. 2022;**182**:110116

[53] Olaciregui-Ruiz I, Vivas-Maiques B, Kaas J, Perik T, Wittkamper F, Mijnheer B, et al. Transit and non-transit 3D EPID dosimetry versus detector arrays for patient specific QA. Journal of Applied Clinical Medical Physics. 2019; **20**(6):79-90

[54] Thongsawad S, Chanton T, Saiyo N, Udee N. Planar EPID-based dosimetry for SRS and SRT patient-specific QA. Life (Basel). 2021;**11**(11):1159

[55] Torres-Xirau I, Olaciregui-Ruiz I, Baldvinsson G, Mijnheer BJ, van der Heide UA, Mans A. Characterization of the a-Si EPID in the unity MR-linac for dosimetric applications. Physics in Medicine and Biology. 2018;**63**(2):025006

[56] Fonseca GP, Johansen JG, Smith RL, Beaulieu L, Beddar S, Kertzscher G, et al. In vivo dosimetry in brachytherapy: Requirements and future directions for research, development, and clinical practice. Physics and Imaging in Radiation Oncology. 2020;**16**:1-11

[57] Rivard MJ, Coursey BM, DeWerd LA, Hanson WF, Huq MS, Ibbott GS, et al. Update of AAPM task group No. 43 report: A revised AAPM protocol for brachytherapy dose calculations. Medical Physics. 2004; **31**(3):633-674

[58] International Atomic Energy Agency. The Transition from 2-D Brachytherapy to 3-D High Dose Rate Brachytherapy: Training Material. Vienna: International Atomic Energy Agency; 2017

[59] Lambert J, Nakano T, Law S, Elsey J, McKenzie DR, Suchowerska N. In vivo dosimeters for HDR brachytherapy: A comparison of a diamond detector, MOSFET, TLD, and scintillation detector. Medical Physics. 2007;**34**(5):1759-1765

[60] Sadeghi M, Sina S, Faghihi R. Investigation of LiF, Mg and Ti (TLD-100) reproducibility. The Journal of Biomedical Physics and Engineering. 2015;**5**(4):217-222

[61] Horowitz YS, Moscovitch M. Highlights and pitfalls of 20 years of application of computerised glow curve analysis to thermoluminescence research and dosimetry. Radiation Protection Dosimetry. 2013;**153**(1):1-22

[62] Pappas EP, Zoros E, Moutsatsos A, Peppa V, Zourari K, Karaiskos P, et al. On the experimental validation of model-based dose calculation algorithms for 192Ir HDR brachytherapy treatment planning. Physics in Medicine & Biology. 2017;**62**(10):4160

[63] Andersen CE, Nielsen SK, Greilich S, Helt-Hansen J, Lindegaard JC, Tanderup K. Characterization of a fiber-coupled luminescence dosimetry system for online in vivo dose verification during brachytherapy. Medical Physics. 2009;**36**(3):708-718

[64] Tien CJ, Ebeling R 3rd, Hiatt JR, Curran B, Sternick E. Optically stimulated luminescent dosimetry for high dose rate brachytherapy. Frontiers in Oncology. 2012;**2**:91

[65] Alvarez P, Kry SF, Stingo F, Followill D. TLD and OSLD dosimetry systems for remote audits of radiotherapy external beam calibration. Radiation Measurements. 2017;**106**: 412-415

[66] Best Medical Canada. MOSFET Products & Accessories. Available from: http://www.bestmedicalcanada.com/products.html.

[67] MOSFET detectors: OncologyMedicalPhysics.com. Available from: https://oncologymedicalphysics.com/mosfet-detectors/.

[68] Tuntipumiamorn L, Nakkrasae P, Kongkum S, Dankulchai P. End-to-end test and MOSFET in vivo skin dosimetry for (192)Ir high-dose-rate brachytherapy of chronic psoriasis. Journal of Contemporary Brachytherapy. 2019; **11**(4):384-391

[69] Melchert C, Soror T, Kovács G. Quality assurance during interstitial brachytherapy: in vivo dosimetry using MOSFET dosimeters. Journal of Contemporary Brachytherapy. 2018; **10**(3):232-237

[70] Phurailatpam R, Upreti R, Nojin Paul S, Jamema SV, Deshpande DD. Characterization of commercial MOSFET detectors and their feasibility for in-vivo HDR brachytherapy. Physica Medica. 2016;**32**(1):208-212

[71] Kumar AS, Sharma SD, Ravindran BP. Characteristics of mobile MOSFET dosimetry system for megavoltage photon beams. Journal of Medical Physics. 2014;**39**(3):142-149

[72] Zilio VO, Joneja OP, Popowski Y, Rosenfeld A, Chawla R. Absolute depth-dose-rate measurements for an 192Ir HDR brachytherapy source in water using MOSFET detectors. Medical Physics. 2006;**33**(6):1532-1539

[73] Therriault-Proulx F, Briere TM, Mourtada F, Aubin S, Beddar S, Beaulieu L. A phantom study of an in vivo dosimetry system using plastic scintillation detectors for real-time verification of 192Ir HDR brachytherapy. Medical Physics. 2011; **38**(5):2542-2551

[74] Therriault-Proulx F, Beaulieu L, Beddar S. Validation of plastic scintillation detectors for applications in low-dose-rate brachytherapy. Brachytherapy. 2017;**16**(4):903-909

[75] Archambault L, Briere TM, Pönisch F, Beaulieu L, Kuban DA, Lee A, et al. Toward a real-time in vivo dosimetry system using plastic scintillation detectors. International Journal of Radiation Oncology, Biology, Physics. 2010;**78**(1):280-287

[76] Beddar AS. Water equivalent plastic scintillation detectors in radiation therapy. Radiation Protection Dosimetry. 2006;**120**(1–4):1-6

[77] Archambault L, Beddar AS, Gingras L, Lacroix F, Roy R, Beaulieu L. Water-equivalent dosimeter array for small-field external beam radiotherapy. Medical Physics. 2007;**34**(5):1583-1592

[78] Chalkley A, Heyes G. Evaluation of a synthetic single-crystal diamond detector for relative dosimetry measurements on a CyberKnife. The British Journal of Radiology. 2014; **87**(1035):20130768

[79] PTW the Dosimetry Company. microDiamond Detector. Available from: https://www.ptwdosimetry.com/en/products/microdiamond

[80] Chofor N, Harder D, Selbach H-J, Poppe B. The mean photon energy ĒF at the point of measurement determines the detector-specific radiation quality correction factor kQ,M in 192Ir brachytherapy dosimetry. Zeitschrift für Medizinische Physik. 2016;**26**(3):238-250

[81] Rossi G, Gainey M, Thomann B, Kollefrath M, Wurfel J, Allgaier B, et al. Monte Carlo and experimental high dose rate (192)Ir brachytherapy dosimetry with microDiamond detectors. Zeitschrift für Medizinische Physik. 2019;**29**(3):272-281

[82] Zhu X. Dosage of radiopharmaceuticals and internal dosimetry. In: Charron M, editor. Pediatric PET Imaging. New York, NY, Springer New York; 2006. pp. 37-46

[83] Maughan NM, Ehtenham A. Current FDA-approved RPTs and their uses. In: Hobbs RF, O'Donoghue J, Clements J, editors. Radiopharmaceutical Therapy and Dosimetry, AAPM Monograph No 40. Medical Physics Publishing; 2023. p. 436

[84] Ross DS, Burch HB, Cooper DS, Greenlee MC, Laurberg P, Maia AL, et al. 2016 American Thyroid Association guidelines for diagnosis and management of hyperthyroidism and other causes of thyrotoxicosis. Thyroid. 2016;**26**(10):1343-1421

[85] U.S. Food & Drug Administration. FDA approves iobenguane I 131 for rare adrenal gland tumors 2018. Available from: https://www.fda.gov/drugs/resources-information-approved-drugs/fda-approves-iobenguane-i-131-rare-adrenal-gland-tumors.

[86] Dauer LT, Williamson MJ, Humm J, O'Donoghue J, Ghani R,

Awadallah R, et al. Radiation safety considerations for the use of $^{223}RaCl_2$ DE in men with castration-resistant prostate cancer. Health Physics. 2014;**106**(4): 494-504

[87] Lehnert M, Ludwig H, Zojer N. Update on the rational use of Y-ibritumomab tiuxetan in the treatment of follicular lymphoma. Oncotargets and Therapy. 2009;**2**:199-208

[88] Hosono M, Ikebuchi H, Nakamura Y, Nakamura N, Yamada T, Yanagida S, et al. Manual on the proper use of lutetium-177-labeled somatostatin analogue (Lu-177-DOTA-TATE) injectable in radionuclide therapy. Annals of Nuclear Medicine. 2018;**32**(3): 217-235

[89] Bolch WE, Eckerman KF, Sgouros G, Thomas SR. MIRD pamphlet No. 21: A generalized schema for radiopharmaceutical dosimetry—standardization of nomenclature. Journal of Nuclear Medicine. 2009;**50**(3): 477-484

[90] Cherry SR, Sorenson JA, Phelps ME. Chapter 22 - internal radiation dosimetry. In: Cherry SR, Sorenson JA, Phelps ME, editors. Physics in Nuclear Medicine. Fourth ed. Philadelphia: W.B. Saunders; 2012. pp. 407-426

[91] Snyder WS, Ford MR, Warner GG, Watson SB. MIRD pamphlet No.11: S, absorbed dose per unit cumulated activity for selected radionuclides and organs. Journal of Nuclear Medicine. 1975

[92] Liu H, Chang JY. Proton therapy in clinical practice. Chinese Journal of Cancer. 2011;**30**(5):315-326

[93] Qiu B, Men Y, Wang J, Hui Z. Dosimetry, efficacy, safety, and cost-effectiveness of proton therapy for non-small cell lung cancer. Cancers (Basel). 2021;**13**(18):4545

[94] Wang LL, Perles LA, Archambault L, Sahoo N, Mirkovic D, Beddar S. Determination of the quenching correction factors for plastic scintillation detectors in therapeutic high-energy proton beams. Physics in Medicine and Biology. 2012;**57**(23): 7767-7781

[95] Goma C, Marinelli M, Safai S, Verona-Rinati G, Wurfel J. The role of a microDiamond detector in the dosimetry of proton pencil beams. Zeitschrift für Medizinische Physik. 2016;**26**(1):88-94

[96] Kerns JR, Kry SF, Sahoo N, Followill DS, Ibbott GS. Angular dependence of the nanoDot OSL dosimeter. Medical Physics. 2011;**38**(7): 3955-3962

[97] Kohno R, Hotta K, Matsuura T, Matsubara K, Nishioka S, Nishio T, et al. Proton dose distribution measurements using a MOSFET detector with a simple dose-weighted correction method for LET effects. Journal of Applied Clinical Medical Physics. 2011;**12**(2):3431

[98] Zullo JR, Kudchadker RJ, Zhu XR, Sahoo N, Gillin MT. LiF TLD-100 as a dosimeter in high energy proton beam therapy—can it yield accurate results? Medical Dosimetry. 2010;**35**(1):63-66

[99] Paganetti H, El Fakhri G. Monitoring proton therapy with PET. The British Journal of Radiology. 2015;**88**(1051): 20150173

[100] Zhu X, Espana S, Daartz J, Liebsch N, Ouyang J, Paganetti H, et al. Monitoring proton radiation therapy with in-room PET imaging. Physics in Medicine and Biology. 2011;**56**(13): 4041-4057

[101] Studenski MT, Xiao Y. Proton therapy dosimetry using positron emission tomography. World Journal of Radiology. 2010;**2**(4):135-142

[102] Xie Y, Bentefour EH, Janssens G, Smeets J, Vander Stappen F, Hotoiu L, et al. Prompt gamma imaging for in vivo range verification of pencil beam scanning proton therapy. International Journal of Radiation Oncology*Biology*Physics. 2017;**99**(1):210-218

[103] Wrońska A, for the SiFi CCg. Prompt gamma imaging in proton therapy - status, challenges and developments. Journal of Physics: Conference Series. 2020;**1561**(1):012021

[104] Draeger E, Mackin D, Peterson S, Chen H, Avery S, Beddar S, et al. 3D prompt gamma imaging for proton beam range verification. Physics in Medicine and Biology. 2018;**63**(3):035019

[105] Panthi R, Maggi P, Peterson S, Mackin D, Polf J, Beddar S. Secondary particle interactions in a Compton camera designed for in vivo range verification of proton therapy. IEEE Transactions on Radiation and Plasma Medical Sciences. 2021;**5**(3):383-391

[106] Rohling H, Priegnitz M, Schoene S, Schumann A, Enghardt W, Hueso-Gonzalez F, et al. Requirements for a Compton camera for in vivo range verification of proton therapy. Physics in Medicine and Biology. 2017;**62**(7): 2795-2811

[107] Schauer J, Wieser H-P, Huang Y, Ruser H, Lascaud J, Würl M, et al. Proton beam range verification by means of ionoacoustic measurements at clinically relevant doses using a correlation-based evaluation. Frontiers in Oncology. 2022;**12**:925542

[108] Assmann W, Kellnberger S, Reinhardt S, Lehrack S, Edlich A, Thirolf PG, et al. Ionoacoustic characterization of the proton Bragg peak with submillimeter accuracy. Medical Physics. 2015;**42**(2):567-574

[109] Lehrack S, Assmann W, Bertrand D, Henrotin S, Herault J, Heymans V, et al. Submillimeter ionoacoustic range determination for protons in water at a clinical synchrocyclotron. Physics in Medicine and Biology. 2017;**62**(17):L20-L30

[110] Yuan Y, Andronesi OC, Bortfeld TR, Richter C, Wolf R, Guimaraes AR, et al. Feasibility study of in vivo MRI based dosimetric verification of proton end-of-range for liver cancer patients. Radiotherapy and Oncology. 2013;**106**(3):378-382

[111] Gensheimer MF, Yock TI, Liebsch NJ, Sharp GC, Paganetti H, Madan N, et al. In vivo proton beam range verification using spine MRI changes. International Journal of Radiation Oncology*Biology*Physics. 2010;**78**(1):268-275

[112] Knopf A-C, Lomax A. In vivo proton range verification: A review. Physics in Medicine & Biology. 2013; **58**(15):R131

[113] Gantz S, Karsch L, Pawelke J, Schieferecke J, Schellhammer S, Smeets J, et al. Direct visualization of proton beam irradiation effects in liquids by MRI. National Academy of Sciences of the United States of America. 2023; **120**(23):e2301160120

[114] Wang CKC. Ch. 3. Progress in Californium-252 neutron brachytherapy. In: Kazushi K, editor. Brachytherapy. Rijeka: IntechOpen; 2012

[115] Maruyama Y, Mesina J, Yudelev M, Wierzbicki J, Deppe G, Porter AT. New

understanding from Cf brachytherapy trials and considerations for neutron therapy of bulky gyn carcinoma for future. Strahlentherapie und Onkologie. 1994;**170**(5):253-263

[116] Peters LJ, Maor MH, Laramore GE, Griffin TW, Hendrickson FR. Review of clinical results of fast neutron therapy in the USA. Strahlentherapie. 1985;**161**(12): 731-738

[117] Catterall M, Errington RD, Bewley DK. Fast neutrons in the treatment of locally advanced breast cancer. European Journal of Surgical Oncology. 1987;**13**(4):315-319

[118] Schwartz DL, Einck J, Bellon J, Laramore GE. Fast neutron radiotherapy for soft tissue and cartilaginous sarcomas at high risk for local recurrence. International Journal of Radiation Oncology, Biology, Physics. 2001;**50**(2): 449-456

[119] Laramore GE, Griffith JT, Boespflug M, Pelton JG, Griffin T, Griffin BR, et al. Fast neutron radiotherapy for sarcomas of soft tissue, bone, and cartilage. American Journal of Clinical Oncology. 1989;**12**(4):320-326

[120] Pelton JG, Del Rowe JD, Bolen JW, Russell AH, Laramore GE, Griffin TW, et al. Fast neutron radiotherapy for soft tissue sarcomas. University of Washington experience and review of the world's literature. American Journal of Clinical Oncology. 1986;**9**(5):397-400

[121] Gordon K, Gulidov I, Fatkhudinov T, Koryakin S, Kaprin A. Fast and furious: Fast neutron therapy in cancer treatment. International Journal of Particle Therapy. 2022;**9**(2):59-69

[122] Suzuki M. Boron neutron capture therapy (BNCT): A unique role in radiotherapy with a view to entering the accelerator-based BNCT era. International Journal of Clinical Oncology. 2020;**25**(1):43-50

[123] Malouff TD, Seneviratne DS, Ebner DK, Stross WC, Waddle MR, Trifiletti DM, et al. Boron neutron capture therapy: A review of clinical applications. Frontiers in Oncology. 2021;**11**:601820

[124] Matsuya Y, Fukunaga H, Omura M, Date H. A model for estimating dose-rate effects on cell-killing of human melanoma after boron neutron capture therapy. Cell. 2020;**9**(5):1117

[125] Rosenfeld AB. Electronic dosimetry in radiation therapy. Radiation Measurements. 2006;**41**:S134-S153

[126] Broerse JJ, Mijnheer BJ, Williams JR. European protocol for neutron dosimetry for external beam therapy. European clinical neutron dosimetry group (ECNEU). The British Journal of Radiology. 1981;**54**(646): 882-898

[127] International Commission on Radiation Units and Measurements. Clinical Neutron Dosimetry, Part 1: Determination of Absorbed Dose in a Patient Treated by External Beams of Fast Neutrons. ICRU No. 45. International Commission on Radiation Units and Measurements; 1989

[128] Burmeister J, Kota C, Maughan RL. Dosimetry of the boron neutron capture reaction for BNCT and BNCEFNT. Strahlentherapie und Onkologie. 1999; **175**(Suppl 2):115-118

[129] Rosenfeld AB, Cutajar D, Lerch ML, Takacs G, Cornelius IM, Yudelev M, et al. Miniature semiconductor detectors for in vivo dosimetry. Radiation Protection Dosimetry. 2006;**120**(1–4): 48-55

Chapter 3

Modern Dosimetry in Radiation Oncology Clinical Trials

Koren Smith, Linda Ding, Maryann Bishop-Jodoin, Matt Iandoli, Fran Laurie, Stephen Kry, Michael Knopp, Mark Rosen, Ying Xiao, Fred Prior, Joel Saltz and Thomas J. FitzGerald

Abstract

Clinical trials in radiation oncology are the best vehicle to optimize our strengths in therapeutic technology, define progress in our field, and improve patient outcome. Trials advance our knowledge in each disease site and provide us information to improve the radiation dose-volume for both tumor control and therapeutic sequelae to normal tissue. An increasing number of systemic and targeted therapies have been developed and are currently in early phase clinical trial design. Ultimately, these new therapies will need to be tested with standard-of-care therapy including radiation oncology. Therefore, during a study, it is essential that radiation therapy is delivered in a uniform and consistent manner for the credibility of the study. If the radiation therapy component of the study does not have a structure or management for maintaining therapeutic compliance, including a real-time data management strategy, it becomes difficult to trust the study outcome and apply the outcome to daily clinical practice. In this chapter, we review the strategy and process involved in the management of dosimetry in radiation oncology clinical trials and how this can impact clinical trial management, primary study endpoints, and the overall success of the study.

Keywords: dosimetry, radiation therapy, clinical trials, cancer treatment, credentialing

1. Introduction

As imaging and therapy technologies have matured over the past 25 years in the field of radiation oncology, the processes of radiation therapy treatment planning and execution have undergone extraordinary change. Accordingly, data acquisition and data management in clinical trials, including radiation therapy, have likewise undergone considerable change commensurate with the technological process improvements in our field. As radiation oncology committees began to develop influence in the National Clinical Trials Network (NCTN), group leadership recognized the need for radiation therapy guidelines to be imbedded in clinical trials and clinical data, including simulation and portal images, to be submitted to a quality assurance (QA) center for review. It was recognized in the early development of radiation oncology clinical trials

IntechOpen

that a system for credentialing institutions and investigators for participation was an important step in ensuring that radiation therapy treatment could be delivered in a consistent manner. In this phase, the Radiological Physics Center (RPC) developed a plan to quantify thermoluminescence dosimetry (TLD) monitoring of each accelerator used for clinical trial participation. Inventories were kept, confirming both the participating investigators and equipment that would be used. As protocols matured and disease-specific protocols required enhanced QA management strategies, the RPC developed a series of phantoms that could be sent to institutions to verify the radiation therapy dose delivered. The phantoms had TLDs imbedded in selected areas for tumor and normal tissue doses. Institutions would irradiate the phantoms and return to the RPC for evaluation. This process would test tumor treatment targeting and image processing in multiple disease areas. The hepatic phantom would also test motion management during therapy. Credentialing confirmed uniform radiation dose execution across centers participating in clinical trials and likewise generated confidence in each institution that therapy delivered at their site was consistent with treatments delivered at other centers. This was important, especially in the early phase of clinical trial development, as computational and quantitative radiation oncology varied between institutions, and establishing a common platform for computation and radiation treatment planning was essential for consistency of treatment execution.

During this era, the infrastructure of radiation therapy treatment planning began a seismic change. For decades, radiation oncology simulation was based on fluoroscopic simulation with planning performed in two dimensions through the isocenter of the therapy treatment field. The ability to perform computations off isocenter was limited and could not be easily adjusted in the care plan. The advent of volumetric radiation therapy treatment planning introduced a new era in radiation therapy treatment planning and delivery of therapy. Computer tomography treatment planning made radiation oncologists and physics planning teams think in terms of volumes treated in three dimensions. The language of radiation therapy moved from calculations measured by isodose lines to dose defined by volume. In this capacity, the importance of imaging in defining the target for treatment became essential and as important a component of QA in clinical trials as uniform computational metrics. The Quality Assurance Review Center (QARC) managed radiation oncology clinical trials for both the adult and pediatric clinical trial groups as well as imaging for the pediatric group. Because of expertise in the collection of planning objects including imaging, QARC began collecting relevant imaging used to define the target for radiation therapy and outcome imaging to confirm the site of recurrence and site of injury when this occurred. In this capacity, imaging could be repurposed as a vehicle to validate disease status depicted on case report forms. The imaging could be reviewed by study and site investigators to ensure that the tumor target was appropriately defined and that treatments were conducted in a protocol-compliant manner. As trials became more complex and digital transfer tools became functional at an enterprise level, the review of objects could be conducted pre-therapy in a real-time manner from anywhere in the world.

This became important for multiple reasons. In what would be referred to today as intermediate and high-risk Hodgkin lymphoma, patients entered on the Pediatric Oncology Group (POG) protocol 8725 were treated with chemotherapy, and half were randomized to receive radiation therapy to all areas of the original disease. The initial publication did not reveal an advantage to those who underwent radiation therapy. However, a secondary analysis of the data was completed by one of the authors (TJF) and demonstrated a 10% statistically significant survival advantage to patients who were treated on study to radiation therapy volumes that were study compliant. Deviations on study with radiation therapy were uniform due to excluding areas of the original disease from the radiation therapy treatment fields, therefore implying that using radiation therapy as a treatment consolidation tool, all areas of original disease need to be treated as part of the treatment planning strategy. This spawned a new approach in the evaluation of radiation therapy treatment plans in cooperative group trials. The initial response in the next iteration of clinical trials involving Hodgkin lymphoma in POG was to move the retrospective review of radiation therapy treatment plans to pre-treatment review of radiation therapy treatment objects to limit deviations and achieve consistency in treatment plans between participating institutions and investigators and limit the influence of non-uniform radiation therapy delivery on the clinical trial design and outcome. Today, clinical trials are managed with real-time and adaptive approaches, including review of radiation therapy treatment plans, using nimble informatics tools that can connect study and site investigators together as soon as digital data arrive at a QA center. Clinical trials today in Hodgkin lymphoma are using informatics tools to augment therapy to those with limited response to induction therapy and titrating therapy to those with rapid response to induction therapy. Advanced stage Hodgkin lymphoma patients on study are now treated with an emphasis on chemotherapy and radiation therapy delivered to areas of incomplete response to systemic therapy as defined on anatomic and metabolic imaging. To achieve the goals of this study, primary and response imaging on therapy as well as radiation therapy treatment objects need to be reviewed at QA centers to ensure the correct areas are being treated to the protocol-compliant dose and the dosimetry meets the study defined constraints to normal tissue. The perception that collecting the data adds to cost and is a burden to site investigators, and there are many examples where limiting data acquisition negatively affected trial outcome and interpretation of the data, leads to unrecovered financial loss and generates a false narrative to trial conclusions [1–8].

The HeadSTART protocol was designed as a randomized study to test the efficacy of adding Tirapazamine to chemoradiotherapy for the management of locally advanced squamous cell carcinoma of the head and neck. Preliminary phase 2 data were favorable, and a phase 3 study was designed to affirm the favorable data of the phase 2 study. The study was designed with on-treatment review of radiation therapy treatment objects (first 3 days of management) and not real-time review to promote worldwide participation on study and facilitate trial accrual. The data management was performed by QARC. Unfortunately, nearly 25% of the patients on study were asked to adjust treatment volumes to ensure protocol coverage of what was interpreted as gross tumor, and of those asked to make changes, less than 50% made the requested adjustment. As a result, the deviations on study significantly influenced trial analysis, and the trial did not reach the desired endpoint. Patients with compliant plans *de novo* had the best outcomes. Those that made the requested changes and those in retrospect who had plans that did not meet dose-volume tumor constraints but thought not clinically meaningful had identical clinical survival outcomes, which were 10% less than those who had compliant plans at the presentation. Therefore, the data make a strong argument for real-time review of objects for study compliance, which can be easily accomplished today with modern informatics tools [8].

RTOG protocol 0617 was designed to test cetuximab with radiation therapy in non-small cell lung carcinoma. Two radiation schemes were imbedded into the study, which included a high-dose (74 Gy) and a lower dose (60 Gy). The study demonstrated no clinical advantage to the higher-dose arm; however, ironically, the local control in the high-dose arm for the first several years on study was 10% worse, and this was statistically significant. Although dosimetry was reviewed and deemed compliant to study metrics, there was no pre- or post-therapy imaging collected on the study. Therefore, the tumor targets and contouring of disease could not be validated, and outcome imaging was not collected to affirm or confirm the site of failure and the relationship of failure to either excluding the disease from treatment or to dose gradient. In this study, cases could be considered compliant to metrics, and the contouring of disease could only be evaluated on the radiation therapy planning systems. Therefore, data acquisition strategies in clinical trials need to include all elements that clinical investigators use to apply therapy to patients in the clinic [9]. The trial must acquire similar information to be confident in the interpretation of the study results. Children's Cancer Group (CCG)/POG protocol 9961 tested the ability to perform both dose and volume titration to children with standard risk medulloblastoma. Important molecular biomarkers were collected as part of the trial design, and this has proven to be invaluable in re-defining risk factors in this disease. Radiation therapy objects were reviewed in real-time. However, in this study, 10% of patients were deemed ineligible for study on retrospective review mostly due to the presence of persistent disease in the posterior fossa post-surgery or evidence of spinal disease not identified at the time of entry onto the study. These patients who in retrospect had a disease at presentation more advanced than study requirement had a significantly worse outcome, therefore establishing the need for real-time review of imaging pre-therapy to ensure the correct patient is entered onto the correct study and the study population is uniform. Each patient on study is a valued resource and deserves our undivided and full attention to facilitate the outcome they deserve [10, 11]. Outcome imaging is essential as it becomes the primary vehicle to assess the level of responsibility imposed by therapy on the location of treatment failure including injury imposed by therapy as well. QARC (now the Imaging and Radiation Oncology Core (IROC), Rhode Island) houses outcome images on Children's Oncology Group (COG) trials, which have been essential in distinguishing disease progression from therapy effect in multiple disease groups, including the central nervous system and late effects imposed by therapy on normal tissue [6, 7].

Therefore, modern dosimetry analysis by members of radiation oncology physics teams works in conjunction with radiation oncologists to ensure contours to both tumor and normal tissue are constructed correctly, and the therapy plan is delivered to protocol specifications and clinical standards to ensure the data can be trusted and applied into clinical practice. In each of these examples, limitations in data and data review as part of the trial design directly influenced the interpretation of the study. Therapy is becoming increasingly complex in both treatment design and treatment execution. Clinical trials currently incorporate the complexities of modern therapy including stereotactic programs, compressed fractionation, radiopharmacy, and particles into trial design and execution. In many studies in pediatric oncology, photon and proton treatment delivery reside synergistically in the study with identical volume guidelines in order to not limit study accrual. In more common adult disease areas, modern physics teams and QA centers will be able to successfully apply strategies for the management of dosimetry on clinical trials for these technologies using the clinical experience of investigative teams [12–20].

2. Dosimetry of modern protocols in radiation therapy

2.1 Qualification

The initial step in the process of evaluation of physics and dosimetry for clinical trials is to visit the IROC Houston website (irochouston@mdanderson.org) to file an inventory list of onsite radiation oncology equipment for treatment planning and delivery. This will include the available equipment for radiation therapy treatment planning, accelerator information, imaging and image validation, and personnel involved in the clinical trial process. This will also identify personnel who will be involved in the clinical trials process including physicians, physicists, and data management staff. IROC will upload the data acquired through the inventory to both the Clinical Trial Support Unit (CTSU) and the Cancer Therapy Evaluation Program (CTEP). As part of this program, all megavoltage photon, proton, and electron beams at each participating site have reference beam output calibration. Brachytherapy audit tools have likewise been developed. If the TLD/optically stimulated luminescence dosimeter (OSLD) measurement is 5% out of alignment, IROC Houston initiates a review process, which will include a review of procedures. If the discrepancy cannot be resolved at this level of interaction, a site visit is performed, which measures calibration, QA procedures, image guidance and multileaf collimator function, and treatment planning system calculations with IROC-measured dosimetric performance [21–23].

These processes ensure confidence that the institution and involved investigators have the equipment and expertise to perform fundamental functions to participate in clinical trials involving radiation therapy and can design and execute patient care in a protocol-compliant manner and meet dosimetry constraints to both tumor and normal tissue targets.

2.2 Protocol development and clinical trial support

Clinical trials remain the best vehicle to move evidence-based knowledge forward and improve clinical care. For the NCTN, IROC becomes involved with study investigators at the time of the concept sheet development. This interaction is particularly important when emerging and developing technologies are being introduced into national and international studies as a structure can be placed into the study to ensure treatment symmetry between institutions, support the development of a uniform study population, and answer protocol-specific questions. This decreases the likelihood that an asymmetric delivery of radiation therapy between institutions will influence the primary study question even when the primary question does not have a radiation therapy study endpoint. During this phase, IROC will develop protocol-specific metrics including tumor target and normal tissue dosimetry constraints to be applied as well as the definition of what would be considered a volume or a dosimetry deviation on study. IROC will write the imaging and radiation therapy protocol guidelines for pediatric and adult cooperative groups for each planned study to make certain the protocol is written in language compatible with the goals and objectives established by the CTEP. The written protocol will include imaging strategies and acquisition pathways for the definition of target and outcome evaluation, radiation therapy dose prescription including percent dose to target volume, protocol compliance objectives and definition of deviations, radiation therapy planning instructions including immobilization strategies and image guidance, QA procedures and implementation, and the data submission process and timing of submission of

Target/OAR—Standard name	Description	Metric	Per protocol	Variation acceptable	Deviation unacceptable
PTV1	PTV1	D95%[%] Dose to 95% of the volume	> 98% of protocol dose	>95% of protocol dose	<95% of protocol dose
GTV_PET	GTV identified on PET scan	D100%[%] Dose to 100% of the volume	> 98% of protocol dose	>95% of protocol dose	<95% of protocol dose
Lungs	Both lungs minus the GTV	Mean[Gy]	≤ 20Gy	≤ 22Gy	> 22Gy
Heart	Heart	V30Gy[%]	≤ 50%	≤ 55%	> 55%
Spinal cord	Spinal cord	D0.03cc[Gy] Max dose to 0.03 cc	≤ 50Gy		> 50Gy

Table 1.
Protocol-required target and normal tissue constraints. The table above shows the expectations of radiation therapy dose criteria for specific targets.

information, especially on studies that permit adaptive volume adjustment based on response to chemotherapy. The formatting also permits patient-specific information including dosimetry to be submitted to Rave and the National Cancer Institute (NCI) Cancer Research Data Commons. Examples of dosimetric guidelines with volumetric language written into studies are listed in **Table 1**. Note that standard nomenclature is required for target and organ names [24].

2.3 Credentialing

For participation in clinical trials involving radiation therapy through the NCTN and the CTSU, the initial step in the process is to contact the IROC Houston office (irochouston@mdanderson.org). A step beyond qualification, credentialing is the vehicle used to determine that the clinical physician/physics team has the resources and expertise to meet individual and specific requirements of a study. IROC implements credentialing through multiple mechanisms that are specific to the clinical trial. Examples include stereotactic therapy phantoms with image guidance including contouring reviews as well as a liver phantom designed to test treatment of multiple lesions with motion management. The phantoms have TLD imbedded into selected areas for validation. Many of the phantoms are technology specific and can be applied across individual protocols and NCI Groups. For example, once an institution passes the phantom for intensity modulation therapy, the credentialing extends to all protocols using intensity modulation across all the NCI Groups. The phantoms can be repurposed for use with varied technologies. For example, the head and neck phantom has been used to credential for intensity modulation and can also be used to credential institutions for proton head and neck therapy. Phantoms have also been made specific to individual disease sites and protocols. For example, pediatric total body radiation therapy and pediatric spine have specific phantoms for participation in clinical trials. The pediatric total body phantom is designed to measure dose uniformity to the target and lung dose. The pediatric spine phantom is designed to test dose across the target in the spinal cord and evaluate dose titration to vertebral bodies largely with proton-directed therapy. The portfolio of phantoms provided by IROC Houston is robust and addresses an important role in the validation of dosimetry for clinical trials. The phantoms are generalizable, and credentialing can be reapplied to protocols once a site has completed the process and is approved for participation in the specific trial.

Credentialing extends into additional evaluations for knowledge assessment. This is very common in industry-sponsored clinical trials. In this circumstance, the institution will receive a case from the QA center and submit tumor and normal tissue contours with a radiation therapy treatment plan that would meet protocol specifications. This process serves an additional purpose of helping site investigators succeed with the data submission process. The data submission objects are reviewed by the QA center. Pre-treatment review of a similar case from an institution can serve as a benchmark case and be repurposed as a surrogate for a knowledge test. Completion of an end-to-end phantom can test all aspects of case development including assessment of the dosimetry of the planned approach to care including image guidance. Once completed and approved, the specific trial can be assured that the institution and identified providers of care possess the skill and have the clinical technology and infrastructure needed to successfully execute treatment for clinical study patients. As technology matures, credentialing becomes of increasing importance in assessing study outcomes. Credentialing for an individual trial can be repurposed and accepted by study investigators at the discretion of the study team and radiation oncology committee members [21–23]. A list of phantoms available for clinical trials is presented in **Table 2**.

2.4 Data acquisition and management

To ensure the quality of the data submitted to QA centers, the IROC process validates that institutions have forwarded accurate and complete information for protocol review. Protocols are complex, and data for individual patients often need to be submitted in sequence for management. For example, intermediate risk COG Hodgkin lymphoma trial AHOD0031 required diagnostic imaging review during chemotherapy to assess response and reassign patients into secondary randomization points based on response to therapy adjudicated by studying anatomic and metabolic

Phantom type (anatomical location of disease)	Modality	Specialized technique being tested
Head and neck (H&N)	IMRT	
Head and neck (H&N)	Proton	
Lung	IMRT	Motion management
Lung	Proton	Motion management
Liver	IMRT	Motion management
Liver	Proton	Motion management
Spine	IMRT/3D	
Spine	Proton	
Head	Stereotactic	Small field dosimetry
Head	Proton	
Prostate	IMRT	
Prostate	Proton	

Table 2.
Partial list of credentialing phantoms available at IROC Houston (irochouston@mdanderson.org).

imaging. Radiation therapy was a tertiary point of randomization based on the completeness of response on imaging. Outcome imaging was also acquired on the study to validate sites of failure and assess toxicity. Therefore, a substantial volume of data had to be acquired over multiple time points over years of participation by each study patient. Patient accrual on this study was 1733 patients. The data provide a wealth of information concerning assessment of disease and therapy response using anatomic and metabolic imaging and are an extraordinary resource for providing structure and imaging guidelines for the next generation of clinical trials in this disease. The success of this study was driven by the processes imbedded in IROC for data acquisition and data management. IROC works to reduce the burden of data submission by providing nimble tools for data submission with data anonymization with continuous improvements to automate the process. IROC uses protocol-specific scripts to perform real-time review of the data, assess completeness of the record, and standardize nomenclature including extraction header and additional identification information from DICOM files. Once submitted, users and members of the QA staff can evaluate and identify gaps in data. The process provides valuable feedback to institutions, which in turn provides an economy of scale for the data submission process and improves trial efficiency.

2.5 Case review

The process of case review ensures that each patient treated on study is cared for in a protocol-compliant manner. The protocol may require treatment approaches that may not fully align with physician preference or department approaches to care; however, the objective is to treat all patients on study in a uniform manner to ensure the study population is treated in a similar manner with respect to tumor dose/fractionation and normal tissue constraints. Although these are specified in the study, contours may be applied differently between institutions and investigators; therefore, the quality review process works to establish common ground between institutional management and study requirements. Imaging has evolved to be an indispensable component to the QA process. Imaging serves many roles in clinical trials. Imaging ensures that the correct patient is entered on the correct study. As evidenced in the medulloblastoma A9961 clinical trial, more than 10% of study participants were not eligible for the standard risk study due to retrospective review of imaging revealing more extensive disease than reported in the primary disease site in the posterior fossa and spine. Similar to asymmetry in the interpretation of response assessment in clinical trials, this has prompted investigators to acquire, manage, and review images in real-time by QA staff and study investigators to achieve the objective of creating a uniform study population including acquisition of outcome imaging to validate clinical outcome including site of failure. Important to radiation oncology and dosimetry, imaging has become essential to the mission for defining target volumes for radiation therapy, and a case review now requires all relevant anatomic and metabolic imaging to be available as part of the review process.

Historically when images had to be copied and data were transferred in hard copy, case reviews could only be performed in retrospect or at best, during the early phase of therapy. This had value, however, even when site investigators adjusted radiation therapy treatment plans in the first week of care at the request of QA review to meet protocol guidelines; patient survival in the HeadSTART trial was 8% less than if the plan met guidelines at the time of data submission. This prompted NCI group leaders and study investigators to investigate pre-treatment and real-time review of imaging and treatment objects to ensure patients on study had protocol-compliant treatment plans and the response to therapy using imaging objects can be validated and is uniform for study interpretation. Tools for digital data transfer for both imaging and radiation therapy today are readily available, nimble, and cost effective. Hundreds of thousands of dollars are lost when patients are deemed study ineligible post-study entry; therefore, making certain the correct patient is part of the correct study improves the confidence investigators have in the interpretation of study outcomes. Although time and experience are needed for institutions and their information transfer teams to be comfortable with digital data transfer and information de-identification, today's real-time review has become a requested standard practice and is available on most studies requiring radiation therapy managed by the NCTN QA centers. Real-time review permits site and study investigators to review plans simultaneously to resolve gaps between site investigators' care plans and study objectives. The process ensures that each patient on study can be treated in a study-compliant manner and that the goals of the study population can be achieved.

Once a study is completed, QA centers continue to collect data on study patients, including completion objects and outcome imaging. This is essential to clinical trial function as outcome imaging is our best vehicle to confirm the status of the patient. Outcome imaging supports our maturation as physicians as we learn to interpret the imprint of therapy on imaging and teaches us how to improve our interpretation of disease progression and therapy effect. The evolving field of artificial intelligence becomes more credible with large datasets to interpret patterns for quantitative analysis. Coupling protocol objects with patient outcome will support the entire oncology community and bring all of us to a broader understanding in applying imaging to outcome analysis.

There is an inherent danger on the horizon with respect to protocol management. There is a perception within studies that too much information and imaging are requested for data transfer to QA centers often hidden under the cloak of "real world" data management. We have sufficient information that too little data collection can lead to study interpretations that are invalid, limiting confidence in the final analysis of the study. The trial data are of vital importance, and limiting data acquisition will contribute to weakening confidence in the results of the trial. It is important to support data collection that is reasonable for the objectives of the study, and if a study has a simple endpoint, a more limited collection of data is reasonable. However, many modern trials ask sophisticated trial questions with secondary and tertiary points of randomization imbedded with response to therapy driving the secondary points of randomization. Trials of this nature require nimble data transfer, with QA centers playing an important role in sharing trial information in real-time between site and study investigators. Although there is a balance between data acquisition and cost, we need to avoid our mistakes of the past in placing a ceiling on data acquisition. The cost is in developing the infrastructure. Once in situ, data transfer is nimble and, in the end, highly cost effective if it improves clinical care.

2.6 Secondary analysis

An important aspect of data collection is to have the informatics infrastructure available to clinical trialists and investigators to ask questions with the data that were not anticipated at the time of trial design. We cannot envision every question before embarking into a clinical trial, and there are moments in clinical trial evaluation, we need to pivot mid-trial as objectives may change based on trial data evaluation and as additional data emerge to help us ask better questions. In this area, data from each of the NCTN Statistical Data Centers coupled with imaging and radiation therapy data housed at IROC are essential to be available both mid- and post-trial for additional analysis and review. In radiation oncology, analysis of acute and late effects from therapy is essential to refining and improving our service to patients. Treatment planning volumetric objects from radiation therapy need to be coupled with outcome imaging to assess dose-volume relationships to outcomes. In this manner, we can assess radiation dose to volume kinetics for toxicity and how the metrics are altered with chemoimmunotherapy. The information gathered on clinical trials is invaluable as the patient population was treated in a uniform format from multiple institutions. Therefore, when analyzed correctly, the data provide information that can be directly applied to clinical care and influence metrics for both tumor control and toxicity in the next iteration of clinical trials. This is an area where QA centers and NCTN data management can support The Cancer Imaging Archive (TCIA) in moving data to the national archive for all investigators to participate and repurpose for research. Data housed in this manner become extraordinary research for projects in artificial intelligence and other endeavors [1–8].

3. Conclusions

Dosimetry is an essential component to the clinical trial process. Quantitative assessment of tumor coverage and normal tissue dose-volume data is the best vehicle to define metrics for tumor control and toxicity. Accurate and uniform dosimetry assessment is crucial to validating clinical trial outcomes. Real-time review of imaging and radiation oncology treatment objects pre-therapy can improve study compliance and secure protocol-compliant dosimetry for tumor targets and normal tissue contours and dose to volume. This generates a uniform study set and serves to limit deviations on study. In turn, the dataset becomes an important platform to evaluate both primary study objectives and secondary objectives not anticipated at the time of trial design. The data on study can be repurposed for multiple studies. For example, the intermediate risk Hodgkin lymphoma study AHOD0031 has generated multiple secondary papers including but not limited to evaluation of the pattern of failure with chemoradiotherapy and interpretation of response to bone lesions as seen on anatomic and metabolic positron tomography imaging. Data are available in nearly all oncology disease sites. Each study has objects that can be repurposed and provides an opportunity to study patients with unusual and exceptional responses to therapy as well as those patients who have biomarkers for therapeutic resistance and progress on primary therapy. These objects can be uploaded to TCIA with clinical information to be used by worldwide investigators for additional studies moving forward. The data are an extraordinary resource, and it remains our responsibility to provide the informatics infrastructure to move imaging and radiation oncology objects for study to a common platform in a public domain linked to pathology and genetic information as a DICOM object linked to the platform in a manner similar to an image. This has the potential of being a worldwide resource for all to learn [25–32].

Acknowledgement

Supported in part by Imaging and Radiation Oncology Core (IROC) Grant, CA180803.

Conflict of interest

The authors declare no conflict of interest.

Author details

Koren Smith[1], Linda Ding[1], Maryann Bishop-Jodoin[1], Matt Iandoli[1], Fran Laurie[1], Stephen Kry[2], Michael Knopp[3], Mark Rosen[4], Ying Xiao[4], Fred Prior[5], Joel Saltz[6] and Thomas J. FitzGerald[1*]

1 UMass Chan Medical School/IROC Rhode Island, Lincoln, RI, USA

2 MD Anderson/IROC Houston, Houston, TX, USA

3 University of Cincinnati/IROC Ohio, Cincinnati, OH, USA

4 University of Pennsylvania/IROC Philadelphia, Philadelphia, PA, USA

5 University of Arkansas, Little Rock, AR, USA

6 Stony Brook University, Stony Brook, NY, USA

*Address all correspondence to: tj.fitzgerald@umassmemorial.org

References

[1] Fitzgerald TJ, Bishop-Jodoin M, Bosch WR, Curran WJ, Followill DS, Galvin JM, et al. Future vision for the quality assurance of oncology clinical trials. Frontiers in Oncology. 2013;**3**:31. DOI: 10.3389/fonc.2013.00031

[2] FitzGerald TJ. A new model for imaging and radiation therapy quality assurance in the National Clinical Trials Network of the National Cancer Institute. International Journal of Radiation Oncology, Biology, Physics. 2014;**88**:272-273. DOI: 10.1016/j.ijrobp.2013.09.030

[3] FitzGerald TJ, Bishop-Jodoin M, Followill DS, Galvin J, Knopp MV, Michalski JM, et al. Imaging and data acquisition in clinical trials for radiation therapy. International Journal of Radiation Oncology, Biology, Physics. 2016;**94**:404-411. DOI: 10.1016/j.ijrobp.2015.10.028

[4] Followill D, Knopp M, Galvin J, FitzGerald T, Michalski J, Rosen M, et al. The Imaging and Radiation Oncology Core (IROC) Group: A proposed new clinical trial quality assurance organization. Medical Physics. 2013;**40**:507. DOI: 10.1118/1.4815652

[5] Fairchild A, Straube W, Laurie F, Followill D. Does quality of radiation therapy predict outcomes of multicenter cooperative group trials? A literature review. International Journal of Radiation Oncology, Biology, Physics. 2013;**87**:246-260. DOI: 10.1016/j.ijrobp.2013.03.036

[6] FitzGerald TJ, Bishop-Jodoin M, Laurie F, O'Meara E, Davis C, Bogart J, et al. The importance of imaging in radiation oncology for National Clinical Trials Network protocols. International Journal of Radiation Oncology, Biology, Physics. 2018;**102**:775-782. DOI: 10.1016/j.ijrobp.2018.08.039

[7] FitzGerald TJ, Rosen MA, Bishop-Jodoin M. The influence of imaging in the modern practice of radiation oncology. International Journal of Radiation Oncology, Biology, Physics. 2018;**102**:680-682. DOI: 10.1016/j.ijrobp.2018.08.028

[8] Peters LJ, O'Sullivan B, Giralt J, FitzGerald TJ, Trotti A, Bernier J, et al. Critical impact of radiotherapy protocol compliance and quality in the treatment of advanced head and neck cancer: Results from TROG 02.02. Journal of Clinical Oncology. 2010;**28**:2996-3001. DOI: 10.1200/JCO.2009.27.4498

[9] Salama JK, Stinchcombe TE, Gu L, Wang X, Morano K, Bogart JA, et al. Pulmonary toxicity in stage III non-small cell lung cancer patients treated with high-dose (74 Gy) 3-dimensional conformal thoracic radiotherapy and concurrent chemotherapy following induction chemotherapy: A secondary analysis of Cancer and Leukemia Group B (CALGB) trial 30105. International Journal of Radiation Oncology, Biology, Physics. 2011;**81**:e269-e274. DOI: 10.1016/j.ijrobp.2011.01.056

[10] Michalski JM, Janss A, Vezina G, Gajjar A, Pollack I, Merchant TE, et al. Results of COG ACNS 00331: A phase III trial of involved-field radiotherapy (IFRT) and low dose craniospinal irradiation (LD-CSI) with chemotherapy in average-risk medulloblastoma: A report from the Children's Oncology Group. International Journal of Radiation Oncology, Biology, Physics. 2016;**96**:937-938. DOI: 10.1016/j.ijrobp.2016.09.046

[11] Packer RJ, Gajjar A, Vezina G, Rorke-Adams L, Burger PC,

Robertson PL, et al. Phase III study of craniospinal radiation therapy followed by adjuvant chemotherapy for newly diagnosed average-risk medulloblastoma. Journal of Clinical Oncology. 2006;**24**:4202-4203. DOI: 10.1200/JCO.2006.06.4980

[12] Withers HR, Taylor JM, Maciejewski B. Treatment volume and tissue tolerance. International Journal of Radiation Oncology, Biology, Physics. 1988;**14**:751-759. DOI: 10.1016/0360-3016(88)90098-3

[13] Emami B, Lyman J, Brown A, Coia L, Goitein M, Munzenrider JE, et al. Tolerance of normal tissue to therapeutic irradiation. International Journal of Radiation Oncology, Biology, Physics. 1991;**21**:109-122. DOI: 10.1016/0360-3016(91)90171-y

[14] Niemierko A. A unified model of tissue response to radiation. Medical Physics. 1999;**26**:1100

[15] Bentzen SM, Constine LS, Deasy JO, Eisbruch A, Jackson A, Marks LB, et al. Quantitative analyses of normal tissue effects in the clinic (QUANTEC): An introduction to the scientific issues. International Journal of Radiation Oncology, Biology, Physics. 2010;**76**:S3-S9. DOI: 10.1016/j.ijrobp.2009.09.040

[16] Marks LB, Yorke ED, Jackson A, Ten Haken RK, Constine LS, Eisbruch A, et al. Use of normal tissue complication probability models in the clinic. International Journal of Radiation Oncology, Biology, Physics. 2010;**76**:S10-S19. DOI: 10.1016/j.ijrobp.2009.07.1754

[17] Darby SC, Ewertz M, McGale P, Bennet AM, Blom-Goldman U, Brønnum D, et al. Risk of ischemic heart disease in women after radiotherapy for breast cancer. The New England Journal of Medicine. 2013;**368**:987-998. DOI: 10.1056/NEJMoa1209825

[18] Kwa SL, Lebesque JV, Theuws JC, Marks LB, Munley MT, Bentel G, et al. Radiation pneumonitis as a function of mean lung dose: An analysis of pooled data of 540 patients. International Journal of Radiation Oncology, Biology, Physics. 1998;**42**:1-9. DOI: 10.1016/s0360-3016(98)00196-5

[19] Graham MV. Predicting radiation response. International Journal of Radiation Oncology, Biology, Physics. 1997;**39**:561-562. DOI: 10.1016/s0360-3016(97)00353-2

[20] Graham MV, Purdy JA, Emami B, Harms W, Bosch W, Lockett MA, et al. Clinical dose-volume histogram analysis for pneumonitis after 3D treatment for non-small cell lung cancer (NSCLC). International Journal of Radiation Oncology, Biology, Physics. 1999;**45**:323-329. DOI: 10.1016/s0360-3016(99)00183-2

[21] Amador C, Keith T, Nguyen T, Molineu A, Followill D. SU-E-P-02: Imaging and radiation core (IROC) Houston QA Center (RPC) credentialing. Medical Physics. 2014;**41**:127. DOI: 10.1118/1.4887940

[22] Followill D, Molineau A, Lafratta R, Ibbott G. The IROC Houston quality assurance program: Potential benefits of 3D dosimetry. Journal of Physics Conference Series. 2017;**847**:012029

[23] Kry S, Molineau A, Kerns JR, et al. Institutional patient-specific IMRT QA does not predict unacceptable plan delivery. International Journal of Radiation Oncology, Biology, Physics. 2014;**90**:1195-1201

[24] Mayo CS, Moran JM, Bosch W, Xiao Y, McNutt T, Popple R, et al. American Association of Physicists in Medicine task group 263: Standardizing nomenclatures in radiation oncology.

International Journal of Radiation Oncology, Biology, Physics. 2018;**100**:1057-1066. DOI: 10.1016/j.ijrobp.2017.12.013

[25] Saltz J, Sharma A, Iyer G, Bremer E, Wang F, Jasniewski A, et al. A containerized software system for generation, management, and exploration of features from whole slide tissue images. Cancer Research. 2017;**77**:e79-e82. DOI: 10.1158/0008-5472.CAN-17-0316

[26] Prior F, Almeida J, Kathiravelu P, Kurc T, Smith K, Fitzgerald TJ, et al. Open access image repositories: High-quality data to enable machine learning research. Clinical Radiology. 2020;**75**:7-12. DOI: 10.1016/j.crad.2019.04.002

[27] FitzGerald TJ, Bishop-Jodoin M, Laurie F, Hanusik R, Iandoli M, Karolczuk K, et al. Acquisition and management of data for translational science in oncology. In: Sundaresan S, editor. Translational Research in Cancer. London: IntechOpen; 2019. DOI: 10.5772/intechopen.89700

[28] Mayo CS, Moran JM, Xiao Y, Bosch W, Matuszak MM, Marks LB, et al. AAPM task group 263: Tackling standardization of nomenclature for radiation therapy. International Journal of Radiation Oncology, Biology, Physics. 2015;**93**:E383-E384. DOI: 10.1016/j.ijrobp.2015.07.1525

[29] Hoppe BS, McCarten KM, Pei Q, Kessel S, Alazraki A, Mhlanga JC, et al. Importance of central imaging review in a pediatric Hodgkin lymphoma trial using positron emission tomography response adapted radiation therapy. International Journal of Radiation Oncology, Biology, Physics. 2023;**116**:1025-1030. DOI: 10.1016/j.ijrobp.2023.02.020

[30] Mauz-Körholz C, Landman-Parker J, Balwierz W, Ammann RA, Anderson RA, Attarbaschi A, et al. Response-adapted omission of radiotherapy and comparison of consolidation chemotherapy in children and adolescents with intermediate-stage and advanced-stage classical Hodgkin lymphoma (EuroNet-PHL-C1): A titration study with an open-label, embedded, multinational, non-inferiority, randomised controlled trial. The Lancet Oncology. 2022;**23**:125-137. DOI: 10.1016/S1470-2045(21)00470-8

[31] Hall MD, Terezakis SA, Lucas JT, Gallop-Evans E, Dieckmann K, Constine LS, et al. Radiation therapy across pediatric Hodgkin lymphoma research group protocols: A report from the staging, evaluation, and response criteria harmonization (SEARCH) for childhood, adolescent, and young adult Hodgkin lymphoma (CAYAHL) group. International Journal of Radiation Oncology, Biology, Physics. 2022;**112**:317-334. DOI: 10.1016/j.ijrobp.2021.07.1716

[32] Castellino SM, Pei Q, Parsons SK, Hodgson D, McCarten K, Horton T, et al. Brentuximab vedotin with chemotherapy in pediatric high-risk Hodgkin's lymphoma. The New England Journal of Medicine. 2022;**387**:1649-1660. DOI: 10.1056/NEJMoa2206660

Chapter 4

Review on Cone Beam Computed Tomography (CBCT) Dose in Patients Undergoing Image Guided Radiotherapy (IGRT)

Panagiotis Iliopoulos, Foteini Simopoulou, Vasileios Simopoulos, George Kyrgias and Kiki Theodorou

Abstract

In image guided radiotherapy (IGRT), cone beam computed tomography (CBCT) is an important tool for patient positioning and verification before treatment. Therefore, the CBCT system has become an essential part and significant component of radiation therapy because it is a development that facilitates more accurate delivery of the prescribed dose to the treatment sites. However, the CBCT system uses ionizing radiation to acquire images for patient setup. Historically, the significance of this imaging dose has been overlooked as it is relatively small in quantity when compared to therapeutic doses used to patients for treatment purposes. In recent years, several works have been made to estimate the dose delivered from CBCT imaging using Monte Carlo simulations in phantoms and patients, thermoluminescence dosimetry (TLD) as well as a variety of other dosimetry methods. The aim of this chapter is to summarize the results from international literature concerning the additional imaging dose delivered to patients due to the usage of Cone Beam CT during radiation therapy, as well as to discuss the future work necessary in order to arrive at a clinically relevant personalized dose estimation protocol.

Keywords: CBCT, IGRT, Monte Carlo, TLD, Dosimetry, radiation therapy

1. Introduction

Cancer even today continues to be recognized as the most lethal among all illnesses [1]. To face cancer, various treatment approaches have been employed in recent years. Alongside surgery and chemotherapy, radiation therapy stands out as a prominent method in cancer treatment. In cases where surgery and chemotherapy are not feasible, radiation therapy becomes the sole available option for certain types of cancer. Considering the crucial role of radiation therapy in the treatment of many cancer types, the accuracy of treatment delivery becomes vital for cancer patients [2]. One of the key factors contributing to the effectiveness of cancer treatment lies in appropriately irradiating the targeted tumor tissue while protecting the surrounding normal tissues as much as possible. Therefore, ensuring proper patient positioning before and during treatment is essential for optimal outcomes [3].

Image guided radiotherapy (IGRT) is an innovative radiation treatment technique that incorporate the use of image guidance which improves the outcome of treatment by delivering the radiation therapy with greater precision to the planned target [4].

In the last decades, patient positioning in radiotherapy relied on the megavoltage (MV) treatment beam and tools like an electronic portal imaging device (EPID) or film positioned behind the patient. However, because of the poor soft-tissue contrast due to Compton scattering a new technique was invested kilovoltage- cone beam computed tomography (kV-CBCT) [5].

Nowadays, the Varian on-board imaging (OBI) and Elekta X-ray volume (XVI) systems are frequently used for kV-CBCT scans during radiotherapy treatment [6]. CBCT has become the most used imaging modality for IGRT and its significance lies in its ability to generate high-resolution volumetric images of patient's anatomy during radiotherapy enhancing the treatment's effectiveness. However, there are concerns regarding the additional radiation dose associated with daily imaging techniques like CBCT [7].

In the past, there was an assumption that imaging doses were insignificant compared to therapeutic doses, leading to less emphasis on reducing them. However, recent changes in imaging practices, involving more frequent exposures, have the potential to accumulate hundreds of mGy doses in patient tissues [8–10]. Unlike diagnostic radiology where imaging settings are often adjusted and optimized for individual patients, this is typically not the case in the context of radiotherapy, where imaging settings remain unchanged and are not fitted to each patient's specific needs [11].

This additional imaging dose delivered to patients from CBCT has become an issue of concern that warrants big attention, so Monte Carlo simulations, Thermoluminescence dosimetry (TLD), and a variety of other dosimetry methods are used to estimate these doses.

The purpose of this chapter is to offer a comprehensive review on imaging dose during IGRT which will provide Medical Physicists and Doctors of a Radiotherapy Department the necessary evidence-based knowledge to plan and execute, in the most effective and safe way, their IGRT treatment.

2. Overview of CBCT in radiotherapy

Cone beam computed tomography (CBCT), is an advanced medical imaging method that utilizes kV X-rays with high contrast. Unlike traditional computed tomography (CT), CBCT uses divergent X-rays, creating a cone-shaped beam. Practically a kV source and a flat panel imager are mounted onto the linear accelerator (LINAC) gantry in a way that they both share a common isocenter with the treatment unit [12].

CBCT plays a pivotal role in modern radiotherapy, serving as a valuable imaging modality for treatment planning and delivery. It provides volumetric images of the patient's anatomy with high resolution, allowing for precise localization of the target area and accurate dose calculation. CBCT offers advantages over conventional imaging techniques, such as the ability to capture three-dimensional images in a single rotation of the gantry and the capacity to monitor anatomical changes during the course of treatment. By integrating CBCT into treatment workflow, radiation physicists and oncologists can optimize treatment plans, ensure proper patient positioning, and make necessary adjustments based on real-time imaging data.

Currently, there are two gantry-mounted cone beam devices. These include the Varian on Board Imager (OBI) from Varian Medical Systems, USA, and the Elekta X-ray volume imaging (XVI) from Elekta Oncology Systems, UK (**Figure 1**). These two systems utilize kV CBCT imaging technology and operating within the range of 30–140 kV. A kV X-ray source (kVS) and a kV detector (kVD) are attached to the linac gantry at a 90^0 offset from the treatment beam.

Megavoltage imaging techniques capture projection images using either electronic portal imaging devices (EPIDs) or, in the case of MVCT in the tomotherapy [13, 14], a single-row CT detector (**Figure 2**). For the EPID technique an AP (anterior/posterior) image is mainly used for 2D positioning and for 3D positioning two perpendicular images AP and lateral are used [15]. Mega voltage CT collects complete 3D images during its 360-degree rotation around the patient [15]. The volumetric MV-CBCT images are reconstructed using EPID projections, leading to a higher dose compared to a pair of orthogonal MV portal images [16]. The imaging dose from a 2.5-MV image (Tomotherapy systems) beam is approximately half that of a 6-MV beam.

KV-CBCT images produce enhanced high-contrast resolution compared to MV-CBCT images. The enhancement in image quality is ascribed to the prevalence of the photoelectric effect at kV energies. On the other hand, at MV energies, the dominant interaction is Compton scattering, which is inversely proportional to photon energy and remains relatively unaffected by the atomic number (Z) of the material. Consequently, the image contrast of MV-CBCT images is reduced for various tissue-equivalent materials [12]. Since the majority of clinical systems use kV CBCT, in the following we will address issues concerning those systems.

The primary utilization of CBCT on linear accelerators (Linacs) is for IGRT but also its capabilities extend to adaptive radiotherapy as well. Highly conformal treatment techniques like intensity modulated radiotherapy (IMRT), volumetric modulated arc therapy (VMAT), and 3D-conformal radiation therapy (3DCRT) necessitate accurate localization of the target and organs at risk. CBCT serves as an advanced imaging modality enabling radiation therapists to correct for target position changes before treatment and monitor complex alterations in patient and tumor anatomy such as weight loss and tumor regression. The advancements in large-area flat-panel detectors and computing capacity have made CBCT the preferred platform for precise three-dimensional IGRT tasks [17]. As a result, it has started replacing

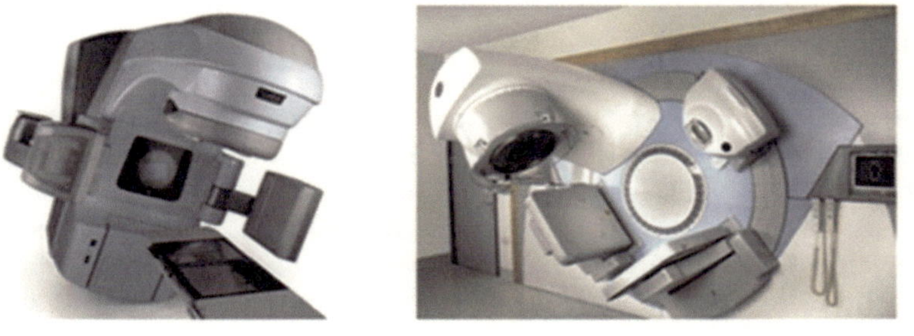

Figure 1.
Cone beam systems. Left: Varian OBI imaging system (courtesy and copyright ©2007, Varian medical systems, Inc.); Right: Elekta XVI system (courtesy and copyright© 2008, Elekta AB (publ)).

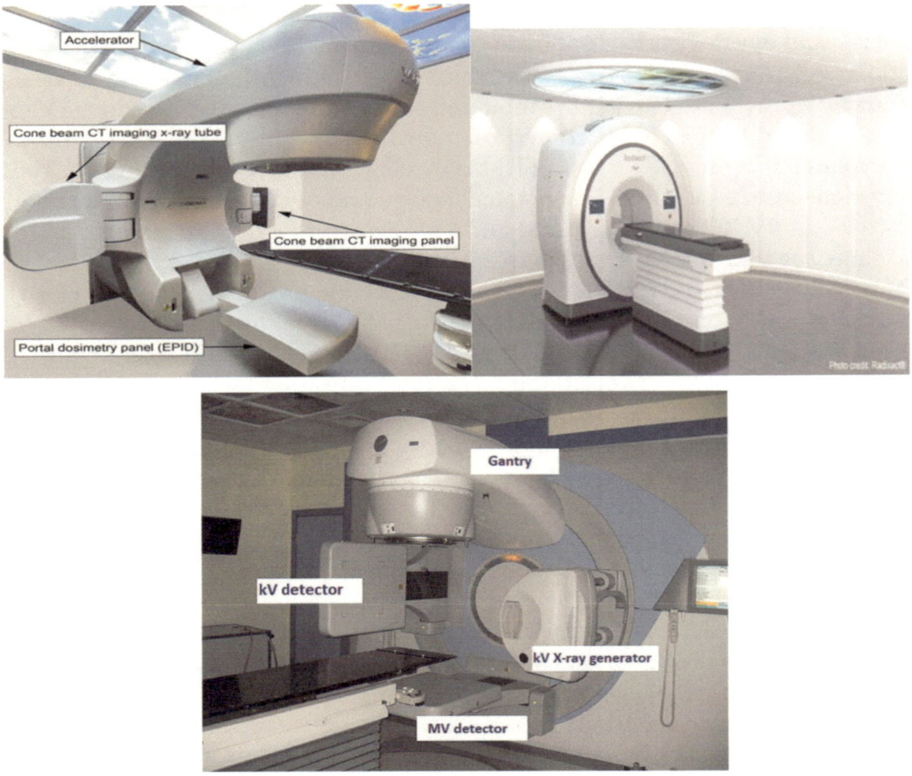

Figure 2.
MVCT systems. UP: Left: Varian true beam Linac (https://physicsworld.com/wp-content/uploads/2020/10/IVD-linac.jpg); Right: Tomotherapy (https://www.parkwayeast.com.sg/tests-treatments/tomotherapy-radiation); Down: Elekta synergy linear accelerator [3].

two-dimensional IGRT to verify if the tumor region remains within the planning target volume (PTV) throughout treatment. CBCT as an IGRT modality has gained popularity for patient setup verification and tumor position confirmation [18] and also the use of CBCT-based IGRT has notably enhanced treatment across various sites [19–21].

The accuracy of delivering the prescribed dose throughout a treatment course using a single reference, known as planning CT (PCT), can be limited by variations in the patient's anatomy, such as weight loss and changes in the size and position of the tumor. Therefore, having information about the patient and tumor anatomy immediately before each treatment fraction becomes crucial for improving treatment outcomes. Adaptive radiotherapy (ART) is a technique that involves modifying treatment parameters, such as field margins and the number of fractions, based on changes observed in both tumor anatomy and patient anatomy. CBCT has the potential to be a valuable tool for online ART [22] because it helps to localize the tumor position in three dimension and detects any changes in tumor or patient anatomy during treatment. This is achieved by fusing CBCT images with PCT images using image registration algorithms and assessing the differences (**Figures 3** and **4**). In cases where it is deemed necessary, the dose distribution can be reevaluated using the treatment planning system (TPS) or specialized software integrated into the imaging

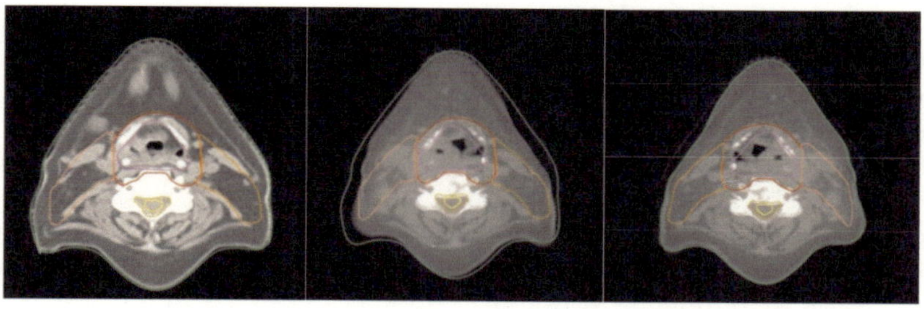

Figure 3.
The PTV and organ outlines were duplicated from the initial CT image (a) to the CBCT image (b) acquired two weeks after treatment. As needed, adjustments were made (c). It is essential to observe the notable alterations in the skin and PTV contours during this process.

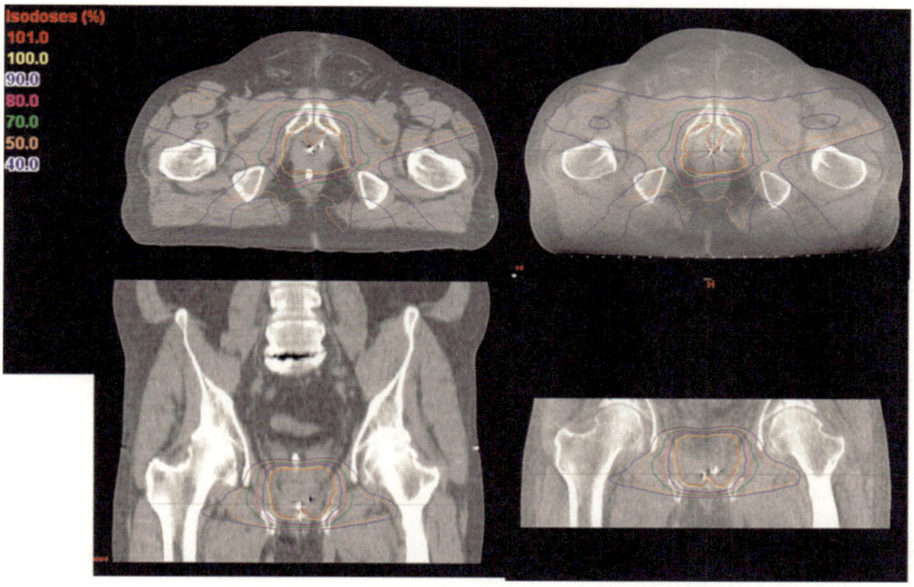

Figure 4.
The dose distributions were computed for the identical prostate IMRT treatment plan using two different imaging sources: The planning CT on the left and a CBCT acquired on the first day of treatment on the right [22].

system. This allows for the generation of optimized treatment plans by incorporating the information obtained from CBCT scans and adapting the dose delivery accordingly [12].

3. CBCT measurements

For CBCT measurements mainly thermoluminescent dosimeter (TLDs) and Monte Carlo codes were used but there are also other detectors such as metal-oxide-semiconductor field effect transistor (MOSFET), ion chamber, radiographic and radio chromic film, optically stimulated luminescence dosimeter (OSLD), and glass dosimeter [8] that have been used, according to literature, for CBCT dose estimation.

Ionization chambers, specifically Farmer-type chambers, are the primary detectors employed for reference dosimetry in clinical settings. These chambers have a small energy dependence across a range of diagnostic and therapeutic energy levels [21]. However, the response of an ionization chamber can be influenced by various factors. These include air density, exposure rate, ion recombination losses, and electric field polarity, all of which impact the collection rate of ion pairs [22]. Reference dosimetry protocols take these factors into consideration to ensure accurate measurements [23].

The American Association of Physicists in Medicine (AAPM) has established a set of guidelines for accurately measuring the reference dosimetry of kilovoltage (kV) energy X-rays [24]. The method involves determining the absorbed dose to water at a depth of 2 cm in a water phantom, and it is calculated using the following formula:

$$D_w = M_{pl} N_k P_{Q,chamber} P_{sheath} \left[\left(\frac{\mu_{en}}{\rho} \right)_{air}^{w} \right]_{water} \quad (1)$$

Where:

D_w represents the absorbed dose to water (Gy),

M_{pl} is the chamber reading, which is corrected for various factors such as ion recombination, polarity, temperature, pressure, and electrometer response (nC),

$N_k$is the air-kerma calibration factor, adjusted based on the spectrum of the X-ray beam used (mGy/nC),

$P_{Q,chamber}$ is the chamber correction factor, accounting for the individual response of the specific chamber used for measurement,

P_{sheath} is a factor related to the sheath used with the chamber,

$\left[\left(\frac{\mu_{en}}{\rho} \right)_{air}^{w} \right]_{water}$ represent the mass energy-absorption coefficients of air and water, respectively [24]. By adhering to this protocol and using the provided lookup tables, accurate reference dosimetry measurements can be obtained for kilovoltage X-ray energies in the specified range.

Several studies have been published regarding the application of optically stimulated luminescence dosimeters (OSL) in medical settings, specifically for therapeutic radiotherapy beams [25–30] and low energy X-rays [31, 32]. The most used OSL dosimetry system consisting of a small reader (microStar) and a detector (nanodot) [33].

The film dosimetry system uses Gafchromic XR-QA2 from International Specialty Products in Wayne, NJ. To scan the films, an Epson Expression 10000XL flat-bed document Scanner is employed by Seiko Epson Corporation in Nagano, Japan. The Gafchromic XR_QA2 film is specifically designed as a quality assurance tool for radiology and dosimetry applications [34].

Thermoluminescent dosimeters (TLDs) are crystalline materials commonly used for radiation dosimetry purposes. Lithium fluoride TLDSs (TLD 100-LiF) are mainly used for dosimetry measurements. To ensure greater accuracy, each TLD is individually calibrated prior to the measurements for certain the photons energy and are irradiated in a poly-methyl methacrylate holder. Subsequently, the irradiated TLDs are read using a Harsaw 3500 TLD reader (Harsaw Thermo Electron, Solo, USA) [3].

The Monte Carlo (MC) method is the gold standard for simulating the tracking of particles and the deposition of radiation doses across various energy ranges relevant to therapeutic and imaging applications. In the context of dose calculations for CBCT imaging, the EGSnrc code system, which consists of the BEAMnrc and DOSXYZnrc codes has been extensively utilized. Additionally, other general purpose MC codes like MCNP and Geant4 have also been employed in this field [8, 35–52].

Dose measurements from CBCT were divided into two categories: in vitro and in vivo measurements.

4. In vitro studies

In vitro measurements in the context of radiotherapy CBCT refer to experimental evaluations conducted outside of a patient's body to assess doses. A significant portion of research on measuring doses from CBCT imaging has been conducted using phantoms [6, 18–44]. The findings demonstrate the wide of doses observed, influenced by various factors such as imaging protocols, phantom characteristics, and dosimeter selection. Understanding these dose distributions is crucial for optimizing imaging protocols, managing patient radiation exposure and ensuring safe and effective radiotherapy treatments [8].

Also, for calculating in vitro patient-specific imaging doses, Monte Carlo code is used and relies on CT images of the unique characteristics of the patient's anatomy. The most precise approach for computing patient dose from diagnostic energy X-rays is through the utilization of the Monte Carlo technique. First, the real X-ray source must be modeled. Using various Monte Carlo codes such as BEAM or GATE, our source is modeled. Therefore, the code must be validated through various procedures

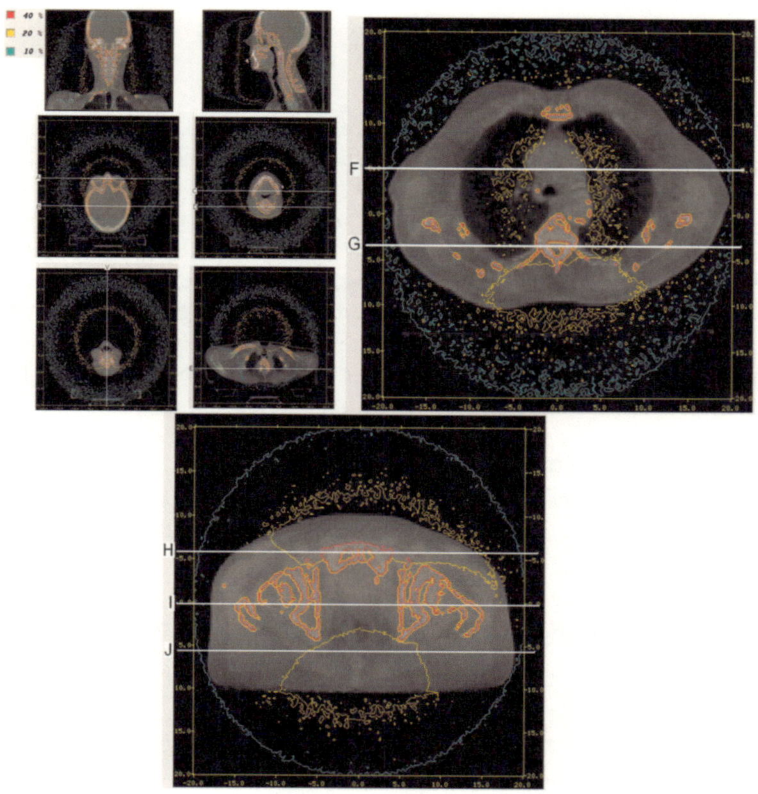

Figure 5.
Monte Carlo isodose lines on reconstructed CBCT image slices for head and neck cancer, lung cancer, and pelvis patient cancer [36].

such as the PDDs and the profiles, and after the identification of the measurements and the Monte Carlo calculated data, our code is validated [36]. The final step is to calculate patient doses with the validated Monte Carlo code using real patient CT images and evaluate the calculated doses (**Figure** 5).

4.1 In vivo studies

To assess the doses received by patients during medical procedures, in vivo measurements can be conducted using available detectors such as diodes, thermoluminescent dosimeters (TLDs), or optically stimulated luminescent dosimeters (OSLDs) [23, 29, 30]. It is important to note that dosimeters designed for in vivo measurements in megavoltage (MV) beams, like diodes, are not suitable for kilovoltage (kV) beams due to the inherent buildup and the significant difference to kV radiation response [51]. In general, patients are typically examined to assess skin dose [52–56]. However, there have been a couple of studies that focused on measuring the dose inside the rectum [57, 58]. The skin dose measurements vary from a fraction of a cGy (for low-dose head and neck imaging) to 7 cGy (for high-dose pelvic imaging), and these measurements depend on the location of measurement, the technique employed, and the patient's size. For the common clinical practice of pelvic imaging using the Elekta system, the rectal dose measurements indicate an average dose of 2–3 cGy to the rectum per CBCT acquisition.

4.2 CBCT doses for different sites

It is crucial to examine the patient doses resulting from CBCT imaging. In kilovoltage imaging, lower dose values are typically observed in head and neck imaging protocols that employ lower time current products (mAs) and partial arc image acquisition. On the other hand, higher doses are found in trunk imaging with higher mAs values and full 360° image acquisition. Megavoltage CBCT imaging results in higher doses compared to kilovoltage imaging, the dose directly correlated to the imaging protocol, specifically the monitor unit (MU) setting used. It is worth noting that kilovoltage doses exhibit greater heterogeneity, typically reaching their maximum value on the skin and showing increased absorption in bone due to the prominence of the photoelectric effect [8].

Table 1 summarizes the results of those studies, encompassing the measured organ doses which range from 0.03 to some mGy per acquisition.

The variation in doses can be attributed to multiple factors, including the type and size of the phantom, the location of the measurement within the phantom, the specific

Manufacturer	Phantom type	Dosimeter/Monte Carlo code	Site	Dose in phantom/ fraction (mGy)	Study
Elekta XVI	Rando	TLD	Head and Neck	0.03–3.43	[3]
Elekta XVI	Rando	TLD	Chest	6.04–22.94	[3]
Elekta XVI	Rando	TLD	Pelvis	2.5–25.28	[3]
Varian True Beam	Rando	Monte Carlo-GATE/Gent4	Pelvis	0.429–37.8	[53]

Manufacturer	Phantom type	Dosimeter/Monte Carlo code	Site	Dose in phantom/ fraction (mGy)	Study
Varian OBI	XCAT	Monte Carlo-GATE/Gent4	Head and Neck	0.29–10.12	[4]
Varian OBI	XCAT	Monte Carlo-GATE/Gent4	Pelvis	3.56–24.13	[4]
Varian OBI	ICRP Computational Phantoms	Monte Carlo-EGSnrc/Beamnrc	Head and Neck	0.27–5.75	[54]
Varian OBI	ICRP Computational Phantoms	Monte Carlo-EGSnrc/Beamnrc	Thorax	0.08–13.79	[54]
Varian OBI	ICRP Computational Phantoms	Monte Carlo-EGSnrc/Beamnrc	Pelvis	0.18–51.38	[54]
Elekta XVI	ICRP Computational Phantoms	Monte Carlo-GATE/Gent4	Head and Neck	0.01–0.66	[55]
Elekta XVI	ICRP Computational Phantoms	Monte Carlo-GATE/Gent4	Pelvis	0.03–34.63	[55]
Elekta XVI	ICRP Computational Phantoms	Monte Carlo-GATE/Gent4	Chest	0.04–21.58	[55]
Varian OBI	Cirs	Chamber/OSL	Chest	2.4–9.1	[56]
Varian OBI	Patents CT images	Monte Carlo-EGSnrc/Beamnrc	Chest	0.35–4.54	[6]
Varian OBI	Patents CT images	Monte Carlo-EGSnrc/Beamnrc	Pelvis	0.14–5.48	[6]
Varian OBI	Rando	Gafchromic	head, chest, pelvis	0.03–2.8 (surface)	[57]
Elekta XVI	Rando	Gafchromic/ XRQA2	Chest	1.2–33.9	[34]
Elekta XVI	Rando	Gafchromic/ XRQA2	Head and Neck	0.9–1.9	[34]
Elekta XVI	Rando	OSL-nanoDot	Head and Neck	0.8–2.1	[32]
Elekta XVI	Rando	OSL-nanoDot	Chest	19.2–22.6	[32]

Table 1.
Summary of CBCT doses.

imaging techniques employed, and the characteristics of the imaging devices. Assigning a single value to represent the dose magnitude based on the imaged anatomy is challenging due to the wide range of experimental setups and variables involved [8].

More specifically **Table 2** shows a comprehensive list of organ doses for different sites.

Organ	Head	Chest	Pelvis
Brain	2.80 [3] - 9.14 [4]		
Eye	1.15 [54] - 2.28 [4]		
Salivary gland	3.18 [3] - 5.64 [52]		
Thyroid	0.89 [54] - 3.23 [3]	1.23 [6] - 10.1 [58]	
Lens	0.97 [55] - 3.43 [3]		
Esophagus	0.18 [55] - 0.73 [3]	1.99 [6] - 7.5 [58]	
Lungs	0.03 [3] - 0.12 [53]	1 [6] - 7.6 [58]	
Spleen		0.6 [6] - 4.4 [58]	
Heart		8.5 [58] - 22.94 [3]	
Skin	0.29 [54] - 9.45 [4]	0.47 [6] - 8.22 [3]	5.4 [54] - 20.9 [58]
Stomach		0.71 [6] - 3.57 [54]	0.13 [55] - 5.18 [3]
Kidneys		0.84 [54] - 23.58 [4]	0.17 [6] - 1.84 [54]
Liver		0.88 [55] - 4.27 [54]	0.12 [55] - 0.61 [54]
Bladder			3.56 [4] - 34.63 [55]
Intestine			0.84 [6] - 24.13 [4]
Rectum			1.27 [51] - 14.4 [4]
Uterus			2.05 [6] - 17.24 [4]

Table 2.
Measured organ doses (mGy).

5. Effective dose

To assess the imaging dose and its biological effect, the equivalent doses to the organs and the effective dose are calculated for each patient during CBCT acquisition. The equivalent doses to specific organs are determined by utilizing the corresponding mean doses and radiation weighting factors. The effective dose, E, is calculated using the equation:

$$E = \sum_{T} W_T \sum_{R} W_R D_{T,R} \tag{2}$$

Where $W_{\square x}$ represents the weighting factor of tissue, W_R represents the radiation weighting factor and $D_{T,R}$ represents the mean absorbed dose to tissue T. The weighting factors are based on publication 103 of the International Commission on Radiological Protection (ICRP) [58, 59].

The AAPM Task Group 75 [15] report emphasized the importance of using effective dose as a metric to evaluate patient exposure to imaging doses. Several studies have reported on the effective doses derived from kilovoltage CBCT utilized anthropomorphic phantoms to measure absorbed does, which were then concerted to effective doses using tissue factors from ICRP report 103. The reported effective dose values for trunk imaging ranged from 1.1 to 24 mSv, while for head and neck imaging, the range was 0.09–9.4 mSv per fraction as you can see in **Table 3**.

	Head	Chest	Pelvis	Study
Effective dose(mSV)	0.289 ± 0.020	1.72 ± 0.07	3.91 ± 0.11	[23]
	0.25	5.56	4.72	[3]
	—	1.06	0.66	[6]
	—	3.9 ± 0.5	15.7 ± 2.0	[58]
	0.09	2.01	7.60	[55]
	2.10 ± 0.08	5.23 ± 0.122	4.89 ± 0.163	[60]
	10.26 ± 0.46	23.56 ± 0.35	22.72 ± 0.29	[60]
	0.04	7.15	3.73	[61]
	1.65	—	8.21	[62]
	9.39	—	16	[62]

Table 3.
Summarized effective doses at different sites.

The wide variation in reported effective dose values can be attributed to factors such as the same anatomical site being imaged, the measured dose, the specific tissue weighting factors used, the imaging protocol (low dose vs. standard dose), and the imager which determines the imaged volume and the use of a bowtie filter.

Typically, when employing low-dose imaging protocols for head and neck imaging, the resulting effective doses are below 2 mSv. On the other hand, standard imaging protocols have been reported to result in effective doses of up to 24 mSv [8].

6. CBCT quality assurance (QA)

To ensure the appropriate dose administration and consistency in medical imaging, it is important to conduct various checks.

To verify the expected imaging dose for each image acquisition procedure which involves a specific protocol the measurement can be conducted in air or within a phantom, as per the guidelines set by the AAPM. To ensure adherence to manufacturer specifications, dosimetry protocols are implemented for kV beams. These protocols are designed to verify that the measured dose falls within the range stated by the manufacturer. The process of acquiring images should encompass the utilization of a specific device. It is important to ensure that the procedures for image acquisition incorporate both the necessary steps. The beam energy should be adjusted to suit the specific application. It is crucial that the energy used is suitable for the desired outcome. In order to ensure that X-ray scattering is fully captured, it is necessary for the sizes to be sufficiently large [16].

It is recommended to utilize the recommendations outlined in AAPM quality assurance reports, including those from AAPM Task Group 142 [63]. Regular consistency checks should be performed annually and after any system upgrades. Moreover, commercially available tools designed for monitoring beam parameters (such as kVp, mAs, etc.) specific to the process can be employed to conduct air-based assessments for imaging dose consistency.

7. Techniques for CBCT imaging dose reduction

Imaging dose reduction is very important and ALARA should be always the most significant principle in practice. As advised by AAPM TG-75 [15] and AAPM TG-179 [63] a, numerous techniques are available to lower the imaging dose to organs at risk [16].

Minimize the size of the imaging field as much as you can. By doing so, the amount of tissue exposed to radiation around the desired area will decrease. Additionally, reducing the top-to-bottom range of kV-CBCT scans can considerably lessen both the overall and scattered radiation dose within the region [64].

Improve the imaging parameters such as kilovolt peak (kVp) and milliampere-seconds (mAs), and choose suitable default clinical protocols provided by the manufacturer for various body areas in typical adult patients (such as pelvis, abdomen, thorax, head, and neck.

Utilizing partial rotation in kV-CBCT scan protocols offers the advantage of selectively minimizing radiation exposure to superficial organs. By employing partial rotation during a head scan, the dose to the eyes (64) can be significantly reduced. This technique can also be applied to decrease the dose to the bladder or rectum during kV-CBCT scans.

Take into account the incorporation of complete bow tie filters during the acquisition of planar kV images. These filters have the capability to substantially decrease both the dose to the skin and the dose to vulnerable organs. It is essential to consistently employ the appropriate bow tie filter for kV-CBCT acquisition, particularly when manual placement of the filter is necessary. Failing to use the filter can lead to an imaging dose increase of 2–4 times [16, 50].

8. Conclusion and recommendations

CBCT has evolved into a conventional imaging method used for patient positioning during radiation therapy. In the past, the imaging dose from CBCT was often disregarded due to its perceived insignificance compared to the therapeutic dose used for treatment. However, the frequent use of CBCT has prompted a reevaluation of the need to measure, document, and account for the imaging dose. This becomes a concern when the imaging dose is substantial compared with the therapeutic dose. In this chapter, the focus is on the attempts to measure and compute the extra dose from CBCT and its potential effects on the total radiation therapy treatment dose [8].

Manufacturers have made improvements in reducing the imaging dose of CBCT units over time, with advancements in technology, modern CBCT systems typically administer lower doses than their older counterparts. Present-day CBCT systems implement diverse techniques, including collimator cassettes and field size-defining blades, to restrict the range of the X-ray beam, which affects the scan volume and the dose to healthy tissues. The use of bowtie filters also influences beam quality and can result in lower skin doses. Additionally, post-processing techniques are often employed to achieve acceptable image quality with lower doses. The magnitude of the dose from CBCT is directly related to the current-time product used in the image acquisition protocol, which can be preset or adjusted by the user. The patient's size, particularly indicated by body mass index (BMI), has a significant impact on the dose delivered at depth, especially for kilovoltage beams. It is noteworthy that CBCT systems typically lack automatic exposure control (AEC) adjustment, a feature commonly found in diagnostic imaging units. However, integrating AEC into CBCT systems would be beneficial in reducing the imaging dose. Additionally, users can employ various techniques to minimize the imaging dose, such as adjusting the start/stop angles of the X-ray source to avoid sensitive organs, using smaller cassettes or field sizes to shorten the scan length, and implementing low-dose protocols to obtain acceptable images [8].

If a protocol with a high dosage is consistently used, the cumulative imaging dose delivered over the course of treatment can be equivalent to a single fraction of the therapeutic dose. In such cases, incorporating the imaging dose into the treatment planning process may be essential. Research indicates that including the imaging dose during plan, optimization can result in a decrease in the total dose delivered to the patient. Nevertheless, this undertaking is difficult and necessitates either employing Monte Carlo simulations or commissioning imaging beams in treatment planning systems. Presently, commercially available systems lack the capacity to calculate the dose from kilovoltage imaging beams. Therefore, it is important to implement the ability to account for imaging dose in commercial treatment planning systems to enable comprehensive dose optimization [65–67].

If the cumulative dose from repeated imaging procedures is anticipated to exceed 5% of the prescribed target dose, it is advisable to incorporate the imaging dose into the overall dose during the treatment planning phase. Estimating patient organ doses can be achieved through patient-specific or non-patient-specific methods. To enable patient-specific imaging dose calculations, it might be necessary to introduce new algorithms for kV beams into commercially available treatment planning systems [62].

As the imaging dose typically constitutes only a small portion of the prescribed target dose, it is deemed acceptable for the uncertainties in calculated imaging doses to fall within 20%. Despite this level of uncertainty, the overall combined dose (therapeutic + imaging) is expected to remain within a range of 2–3% [62].

This chapter highlights the increasing awareness and interest in evaluating the additional dose from CBCT. As image guidance plays a vital role in radiation therapy treatment, and with the possibility of treatment adaptation based on dose recalculation in the patient's actual treatment position, it is crucial to implement tools for controlling and managing the potential negative effects of the extra dose arising from on-board imaging devices.

In the future, there should be some protocol according to which it will be practically possible to be able to calculate for each patient their imaging dose from the CBCT so that there is an individualized integrated view of the total dose (treatment and imaging) of the patient.

Conflict of interest

The authors declare no conflict of interest.

Author details

Panagiotis Iliopoulos[1]*, Foteini Simopoulou[2], Vasileios Simopoulos[2], George Kyrgias[2] and Kiki Theodorou[1]

1 Faculty of Medicine, Medical Physics Department, University of Thessaly, Larisa, Greece

2 Faculty of Medicine, Radiotherapy Department, University of Thessaly, Larisa, Greece

*Address all correspondence to: Iliopoulos_panagiotis@hotmail.com

References

[1] Stewart BW, Wild C. International Agency for Research on Cancer. World Cancer Report. France: Lyon CEDEX; 2014. p. 2014

[2] Xu XG, Bednarz B, Paganetti H. A review of dosimetry studies on external-beam radiation treatment with respect to second cancer induction. Physics in Medicine and Biology. 2008; **53**(13):R193

[3] Özseven A, Dirican B. Evaluation of patient organ doses from kilovoltage cone-beam CT imaging in radiation therapy. Reports of Practical Oncology and Radiotherapy. 2021;**26**(2):251-258

[4] Son K, Kim JS, Lee H, Cho S. Imaging dose of human organs from kV-CBCT in image-guided radiation therapy. Radiation Protection Dosimetry. 2017; **175**(2):194-200

[5] Buckley JG, Wilkinson D, Malaroda A, Metcalfe P. Investigation of the radiation dose from cone-beam CT for image-guided radiotherapy: A comparison of methodologies. Journal of Applied Clinical Medical Physics. 2018; **19**(1):174-183

[6] Abuhaimed A, Martin CJ. Assessment of organ and size-specific effective doses from cone beam CT (CBCT) in image-guided radiotherapy (IGRT) based on body mass index (BMI). Radiation Physics and Chemistry. 2023;**208**: 110889

[7] Cumur C, Fujibuchi T, Hamada K. Dose estimation for cone-beam computed tomography in image-guided radiation therapy using mesh-type reference computational phantoms and assuming head and neck cancer. Journal of Radiological Protection. 2022;**42**(2): 021533

[8] Alaei P, Spezi E. Imaging dose from cone beam computed tomography in radiation therapy. Physica Medica. 2015; **31**(7):647-658

[9] Zhou L, Bai S, Zhang Y, Ming X, Deng J. Imaging dose and cancer risk in image guided radiation therapy of cancers. International Journal of Radiation Oncology Biology Physics. 2015;**93**(3):S181-S182

[10] Deng J, Zhang Y, Zhou L, Ming X, Wu H. Why are we concerned about imaging dose in the radiotherapy of cancers? Austin Journal of Radiology. 2014;**1**:1-3

[11] Martin C, Kron T, Vassileva J, Wood T, Joyce C, Ung N, et al. An international survey of imaging practices in radiotherapy. Physica Medica. 2021; **90**:53-65

[12] Srinivasan K, Mohammadi M, Shepherd J. Applications of linac-mounted kilovoltage cone-beam computed tomography in modern radiation therapy: A review. Polish Journal of Radiology. 2014;**79**:181

[13] Mackie TR, Kapatoes J, Ruchala K, Lu W, Wu C, Olivera G, et al. Image guidance for precise conformal radiotherapy. International Journal of Radiation Oncology Biology Physics. 2003;**56**(1):89-105

[14] Mackie TR, Balog J, Ruchala K, Shepard D, Aldridge S, Fitchard E, et al. Tomotherapy. Seminars Radiation Oncology. Jan 1999;**9**(1):108-117

[15] Murphy MJ, Balter J, Balter S, BenComo JA Jr, Das IJ, Jiang SB, et al. The management of imaging dose during image-guided radiotherapy: Report of

the AAPM task group 75. Medical Physics. 2007;**34**(10):4041-4063

[16] Ding GX, Alaei P, Curran B, Flynn R, Gossman M, Mackie TR, et al. Image guidance doses delivered during radiotherapy: Quantification, management, and reduction: Report of the AAPM therapy physics committee task group 180. Medical Physics. 2018; **45**(5):e84-e99

[17] Jaffray DA, Siewerdsen JH, Wong JW, Martinez AA. Flat-panel cone-beam computed tomography for image-guided radiation therapy. International Journal of Radiation Oncology Biology Physics. 2002;**53**(5): 1337-1349

[18] Moore CJ, Amer A, Marchant T, Sykes JR, Davies J, Stratford J, et al. Developments in and experience of kilovoltage X-ray cone beam image-guided radiotherapy. The British Journal of Radiology. 2006;**79**(special_issue_1): S66-S78

[19] Oldham M, Létourneau D, Watt L, Hugo G, Yan D, Lockman D, et al. Cone-beam-CT guided radiation therapy: A model for on-line application. Radiotherapy and Oncology. 2005;**75**(3): 271-2E1

[20] Guckenberger M, Meyer J, Wilbert J, Baier K, Sauer O, Flentje M. Precision of image-guided radiotherapy (IGRT) in six degrees of freedom and limitations in clinical practice. Strahlentherapie und Onkologie. Jun 2007;**183**(6):307-313

[21] Boda-Heggemann J, Lohr F, Wenz F, Flentje M, Guckenberger M. kV-Cone-beam-CT-basierte bildgeführte Strahlentherapie–ein klinischer Überblick: A Clinical Review. Strahlentherapie und Onkologie. 2011; **187**:284-291

[22] Ding GX, Duggan DM, Coffey CW, Deeley M, Hallahan DE, Cmelak A, et al. A study on adaptive IMRT treatment planning using kV cone-beam CT. Radiotherapy and Oncology. 2007;**85**(1): 116-125

[23] Gilling L. A GATE Monte Carlo Dose Analysis from Varian XI Cone-beam Computed Tomography. University of Canterbury; 2019

[24] Ma CM. AAPM TG-61 report on kilovoltage X-ray dosimetry: Formalisms and applications. In: Proceedings of the 22nd Annual International Conference of the IEEE Engineering in Medicine and Biology Society (Cat. No.00CH37143), Chicago, IL, USA. 2000. Vol. 3. pp. 2308-2312. DOI: 10.1109/IEMBS.2000.900604

[25] Schembri V, Heijmen B. Optically stimulated luminescence (OSL) of carbon-doped aluminum oxide for film dosimetry in radiotherapy. Medical Physics. 2007;**34**(6Part1):2113-2118

[26] Jursinic PA. Characterization of optically stimulated luminescent dosimeters, OSLDs, for clinical dosimetric measurements. Medical Physics. 2007;**34**(12):4594-4604

[27] Yukihara E, McKeever S. Optically stimulated luminescence (OSL) dosimetry in medicine. Physics in Medicine and Biology. 2008;**53**(20):R351

[28] Jursinic PA. Changes in optically stimulated luminescent dosimeter (OSLD) dosimetric characteristics with accumulated dose. Medical Physics. 2010;**37**(1):132-140

[29] Mrčela I, Bokulić T, Izewska J, Budanec M, Fröbe A, Kusić Z. Optically stimulated luminescence in vivo dosimetry for radiotherapy: Physical characterization and clinical

measurements in 60Co beams. Physics in Medicine and Biology. 2011;**56**(18):6065

[30] Reft CS. The energy dependence and dose response of a commercial optically stimulated luminescent detector for kilovoltage photon, megavoltage photon, and electron, proton, and carbon beams. Medical Physics. 2009;**36**(5):1690-1699

[31] Al-Senan RM, Hatab MR. Characteristics of an OSLD in the diagnostic energy range. Medical Physics. 2011;**38**(7):4396-4405

[32] Ding GX, Malcolm AW. An optically stimulated luminescence dosimeter for measuring patient exposure from imaging guidance procedures. Physics in Medicine and Biology. 2013;**58**(17):5885

[33] Mail N, Yusuf M, Alothmany N, Kinsara AA, Abdulkhaliq F, Ghamdi SM, et al. A methodology for on-board CBCT imaging dose using optically stimulated luminescence detectors. Journal of Applied Clinical Medical Physics. 2016; **17**(5):482-499

[34] Giaddui T, Cui Y, Galvin J, Yu Y, Xiao Y. Comparative dose evaluations between XVI and OBI cone beam CT systems using Gafchromic XRQA2 film and nanoDot optical stimulated luminescence dosimeters. Medical Physics. 2013;**40**(6Part1):062102

[35] Ding GX, Coffey CW. Beam characteristics and radiation output of a kilovoltage cone-beam CT. Physics in Medicine and Biology. 2010;**55**(17):5231

[36] Ding GX, Duggan DM, Coffey CW. Accurate patient dosimetry of kilovoltage cone-beam CT in radiation therapy. Medical Physics. 2008;**35**(3): 1135-1144

[37] Spezi E, Downes P, Radu E, Jarvis R. Monte Carlo simulation of an x-ray volume imaging cone beam CT unit. Medical Physics. 2009;**36**(1):127-136

[38] Downes P, Jarvis R, Radu E, Kawrakow I, Spezi E. Monte Carlo simulation and patient dosimetry for a kilovoltage cone-beam CT unit. Medical Physics. 2009;**36**(9Part1):4156-4167

[39] Chow JC, Leung MK, Islam MK, Norrlinger BD, Jaffray DA. Evaluation of the effect of patient dose from cone beam computed tomography on prostate IMRT using Monte Carlo simulation. Medical Physics. 2008;**35**(1):52-60

[40] Deng J, Chen Z, Roberts KB, Nath R. Kilovoltage imaging doses in the radiotherapy of pediatric cancer patients. International Journal of Radiation Oncology Biology Physics. 2012;**82**(5):1680-1688

[41] Deng J, Chen Z, James BY, Roberts KB, Peschel RE, Nath R. Testicular doses in image-guided radiotherapy of prostate cancer. International Journal of Radiation Oncology Biology Physics. 2012; **82**(1):e39-e47

[42] Gu J, Bednarz B, Xu XG, Jiang SB. Assessment of patient organ doses and effective doses using the VIP-man adult male phantom for selected cone-beam CT imaging procedures during image guided radiation therapy. Radiation Protection Dosimetry. 2008;**131**(4):431-443

[43] Walters B, Ding G, Kramer R, Kawrakow I. Skeletal dosimetry in cone beam computed tomography. Medical Physics. 2009;**36**(7):2915-2922

[44] Ding GX, Coffey CW. Radiation dose from kilovoltage cone beam computed tomography in an image-guided radiotherapy procedure. International Journal of Radiation Oncology Biology Physics. 2009;**73**(2): 610-617

[45] Ding A, Gu J, Trofimov AV, Xu XG. Monte Carlo calculation of imaging doses from diagnostic multidetector CT and kilovoltage cone-beam CT as part of prostate cancer treatment plans. Medical Physics. 2010;**37**(12):6199-6204

[46] Qiu Y, Popescu I, Duzenli C, Moiseenko V. Mega-voltage versus kilo-voltage cone beam CT used in image guided radiation therapy: Comparative study of microdosimetric properties. Radiation Protection Dosimetry. 2011; **143**(2–4):477-480

[47] Spezi E, Downes P, Jarvis R, Radu E, Staffurth J. Patient-specific three-dimensional concomitant dose from cone beam computed tomography exposure in image-guided radiotherapy. International Journal of Radiation Oncology Biology Physics. 2012;**83**(1): 419-426

[48] Qiu Y, Moiseenko V, Aquino-Parsons C, Duzenli C. Equivalent doses for gynecological patients undergoing IMRT or RapidArc with kilovoltage cone beam CT. Radiotherapy and Oncology. 2012;**104**(2):257-262

[49] Zhang Y, Yan Y, Nath R, Bao S, Deng J. Personalized assessment of kV cone beam computed tomography doses in image-guided radiotherapy of pediatric cancer patients. International Journal of Radiation Oncology Biology Physics. 2012;**83**(5): 1649-1654

[50] Ding GX, Munro P. Radiation exposure to patients from image guidance procedures and techniques to reduce the imaging dose. Radiotherapy and Oncology. 2013;**108**(1):91-98

[51] Son K, Cho S, Kim JS, Han Y, Ju SG, Choi DH. Evaluation of radiation dose to organs during kilovoltage cone-beam computed tomography using Monte Carlo simulation. Journal of Applied Clinical Medical Physics. 2014;**15**(2): 295-302

[52] Spezi E, Volken W, Frei D, Fix M. A virtual source model for kilo-voltage cone beam CT: Source characteristics and model validation. Medical Physics. 2011;**38**(9):5254-5263

[53] Gilling L, Ali O. Organ dose from Varian XI and Varian OBI systems are clinically comparable for pelvic CBCT imaging. Physical and Engineering Sciences in Medicine. 2022;**45**(1):279-285

[54] Abuhaimed A, Martin CJ, Sankaralingam M. A Monte Carlo study of organ and effective doses of cone beam computed tomography (CBCT) scans in radiotherapy. Journal of Radiological Protection. 2017;**38**(1):61

[55] Marchant TE, Joshi KD. Comprehensive Monte Carlo study of patient doses from cone-beam CT imaging in radiotherapy. Journal of Radiological Protection. 2016;**37**(1):13

[56] Winey B, Zygmanski P, Lyatskaya Y. Evaluation of radiation dose delivered by cone beam CT and tomosynthesis employed for setup of external breast irradiation. Medical Physics. 2009;**36**(1): 164-173

[57] Tomic N, Devic S, DeBlois F, Seuntjens J. Reference radiochromic film dosimetry in kilovoltage photon beams during CBCT image acquisition. Medical Physics. 2010;**37**(3):1083-1092

[58] Yuasa Y, Shiinoki T, Onizuka R, Fujimoto K. Estimation of effective imaging dose and excess absolute risk of secondary cancer incidence for four-dimensional cone-beam computed tomography acquisition. Journal of Applied Clinical Medical Physics. 2019; **20**(11):57-68

[59] Protection R. ICRP publication 103. Annals of the ICRP. 2007;**37**(2.4):2

[60] Kan MW, Leung LH, Wong W, Lam N. Radiation dose from cone beam computed tomography for image-guided radiation therapy. International Journal of Radiation Oncology Biology Physics. 2008;**70**(1):272-279

[61] Hyer DE, Serago CF, Kim S, Li JG, Hintenlang DE. An organ and effective dose study of XVI and OBI cone-beam CT systems. Journal of Applied Clinical Medical Physics. 2010; **11**(2):181-197

[62] Cheng HC, Wu VW, Liu ES, Kwong DL. Evaluation of radiation dose and image quality for the Varian cone beam computed tomography system. International Journal of Radiation Oncology Biology Physics. 2011;**80**(1): 291-300

[63] Bissonnette J, Balter PA, Dong L, Langen KM, Lovelock DM, Miften M, et al. Quality assurance for image-guided radiation therapy utilizing CT-based technologies: A report of the AAPM TG-179. Medical Physics. 2012;**39**(4): 1946-1963

[64] Ding GX, Munro P, Pawlowski J, Malcolm A, Coffey CW. Reducing radiation exposure to patients from kV-CBCT imaging. Radiotherapy and Oncology. 2010;**97**(3):585-592

[65] Miften M, Gayou O, Reitz B, Fuhrer R, Leicher B, Parda DS. IMRT planning and delivery incorporating daily dose from mega-voltage cone-beam computed tomography imaging. Medical Physics. 2007;**34**(10): 3760-3767

[66] Alaei P, Spezi E, Reynolds M. Dose calculation and treatment plan optimization including imaging dose from kilovoltage cone beam computed tomography. Acta Oncologica. 2014; **53**(6):839-844

[67] Grelewicz Z, Wiersma RD. Combined MV + kV inverse treatment planning for optimal kV dose incorporation in IGRT. Physics in Medicine and Biology. 2014;**59**(7):1607

Section 2

New Trends in Radiopharmaceuticals

Chapter 5

Recent Advances of Copper-64 Based Radiopharmaceuticals in Nuclear Medicine

Nasim Vahidfar, Mohsen Bakhshi Kashi, Saeed Afshar, Peyman Sheikhzadeh, Saeed Farzanefar, Yalda Salehi, Ebrahim Delpasand, Eóin N. Molloy, Siroos Mirzaei, Hojjat Ahmadzadehfar and Elisabeth Eppard

Abstract

Copper radioisotopes including copper-60/61/62, and -64 exhibit a wide range of decay characteristics, making them appropriate choices for diagnostic/therapeutic (theranostic) applications in nuclear medicine. One notable feature of copper is the feasible coordination chemistry, which makes radiolabeling of a wide range of chemical structures including antibodies, proteins, peptides, and other biologically relevant small molecules possible. This chapter will summarize common radiopharmaceuticals of copper-64 and their radiation dosimetry in order to highlight recent improvements of positron emission tomography diagnostics.

Keywords: copper-64, radiopharmaceuticals, medical imaging, positron emission tomography, oncology

1. Introduction

Targeted nuclear imaging has significantly improved modern diagnostic methods and therapeutic procedures [1] by allowing for better imaging contrast, enhanced therapy effectivity, and reduction of radiation dose to the patients [2, 3]. Several classes of substances, including endogenous biomolecules, exogenous natural products, and synthetic molecules can be used practically as molecular probes for imaging or therapy [1]. Typically, molecular imaging is considered as a revolution in association with diagnosis and monitoring of disease [4]. Currently, positron emission tomography/computed tomography (PET/CT), alongside other diagnostic modalities, is well established, particularly given advances of PET/CT in terms of its superior resolution, sensitivity, and imaging quantification. These characteristics have made PET/CT a preferred method for molecular imaging [5–7]. In particular, copper radioisotopes have attracted much attention among PET radionuclides [8, 9]. Copper is an essential trace element in all living organisms [10–13]. The available radioisotopes of copper, including copper-60 (60Cu), copper-61 (61Cu), copper-62 (62Cu), and copper-64 (64Cu), are appropriate for molecular imaging/or therapeutic applications (**Table 1**) [14].

With a wide range of half-lives extending from 9.7 min to 12.7 h, copper provides a series of radioisotopes suited for diagnostic or therapeutic applications in nuclear medicine [13, 15]. Copper coordination chemistry has the ability to form complex compounds with many ligands including antibodies, peptides, proteins, and other relevant small molecules [14, 16]. The long half-life of $^{64/67}Cu$ allows for sufficient accumulation of radiolabeled compounds in targeted organs, specific and proper uptake and, as a result, considerably higher contrast and image quality [14]. Each of the above-mentioned copper-based radioisotopes has variably preferable properties based on given applications. For example, the shorter half-life and higher positron decay fraction of copper-60 and -62 make them ideal radionuclides for imaging evaluation of radiotracers with faster pharmacokinetic procedures such as radiolabeled small molecules. In contrast, the longer half-life of ^{64}Cu would be appropriate for radiolabeling of chemical structures, in order to formulate radiopharmaceuticals with slower pharmacokinetics, including radiolabeled peptides, nanoparticles, monoclonal antibodies (mAbs), antibodies, and higher molecular weight polypeptides [14]. While all copper radioisotopes are currently used in clinical applications, ^{64}Cu has shown the most promising results in both preclinical and clinical studies [16]. In particular, the longer half-life of ^{64}Cu (12.7 h) allows for the extension of the imaging period, which in turn compensates for lower sensitivity [9]. In a study assessing resolution, the "Derenzo" phantom application, demonstrated that PET imaging qualities with ^{64}Cu are accurately comparable to fluorine-18 (^{18}F) [17]. As ^{64}Cu-radiopharmaceuticals for the evaluation of human morbidities are currently undergoing significant developments [18], this chapter will focus on ^{64}Cu-radiopharmaceuticals that have been already approved for clinical trials or are close to being transferred to clinical settings (**Table 2**).

Radioisotope	Half-life ($T_{1/2}$)	Decay mode (abundance %)	Energy (keV)	Source	Application
^{60}Cu	23.7 min	β^+ (93)	2940,3920	Cyclotron	Imaging
		γ (7)	511-467-826-1332		
^{61}Cu	3.3 h	β^+ (60)	1220,1159	Cyclotron	Imaging
		γ (40)	511-283-589-656		
^{62}Cu	9.7 min	β^+ (98)	2925	Cyclotron	Imaging
		γ (2)	511	Generator	
^{64}Cu	12.7 h	β^+ (19)	657	Cyclotron	Imaging/ Therapy
		γ (43)	511-1346		
		β^- (38.4)	573		
^{67}Cu	2.58 d	β^- (100)	575	Cyclotron	Therapy

Table 1.
Physical characterization of copper radioisotopes [11]. β = Beta decay, γ = Gamma decay.

	Radiopharmaceuticals	Condition or disease	Phase	Last update posted
^{60}Cu	—	—	—	—
^{61}Cu	—	—	—	—
^{62}Cu	[^{62}Cu]Cu-ethylglyoxal bis (thiosemicarbazone)	Renal failure	2	April, 2017 (Terminated)
^{64}Cu	[^{64}Cu]Cu-ATSM	Rectal cancer	2	May, 2021
		Cervical cancer	2	February, 2021
		NSCLC	N/A	July, 2013
	[^{64}Cu]Cu-DOTA-TATE	Neuroendocrine tumors	3	July, 2019 (Approved for marketing)
	[^{64}Cu]Cu-DOTA-alendronate	Breast carcinoma	Early 1	November, 2021
	[^{64}Cu] Cu-DOTA-trastuzumab	Gastric cancer	N/A	March, 2021
		Breast cancer	N/A	January, 2021
	[^{64}Cu]Cu-Rituximab	Non-Hodgkin's lymphoma	N/A	October, 2016
	[^{64}Cu]Cu-DOTA-ECL1i	Head and neck cancer	1	December, 2021
	[^{64}Cu]Cu-LLP2A	Multiple myeloma	Early 1	August, 2021
	[^{64}Cu]Cu-SARTATE	Neuroendocrine tumors	2	May, 2021
	[^{64}Cu]Cu-SAR-bisPSMA	Prostatic neoplasms	1	August, 2021
	[^{64}Cu]Cu-DOTA-TLX592	Metastatic prostate cancer	Early 1	August, 2021
	[^{64}Cu] Cu-DOTA-pembrolizumab	Hematopoietic and lymphoid cell neoplasm	1	November, 2021
	[^{64}Cu]Cu-Macrin			
	[^{64}Cu]Cu-NOTA-PSMAi-PEG-Cy5.5-C′ dots	Sarcoid	1	September, 2021
	[^{64}Cu]Cu-FBP8	Prostate cancer	1	September, 2021
		Pulmonary embolism	1	July, 2019

Table 2.
^{64}Cu radiopharmaceuticals list entered in clinical trials.

1.1 ^{64}Cu radiopharmaceuticals and their role in clinical studies

As it described above, ^{64}Cu is a promising radionuclide that can be incorporated into many bio-conjugated chemical structures to further develop diagnostic and therapeutic agents with specific oncological indications [19]. The intermediate half-life of copper-64 (12.7 h) and its' short positron range (comparable to fluorine-18) allow ^{64}Cu to create high-resolution PET tracers [20, 21]. Hypoxia imaging agents based on bis(thiosemicarbazone) complexes radiolabeled with ^{64}Cu have been used successfully for PET imaging of various types of tumors [22–24], blood flow [25], disease related to metabolism alterations [26–29], and cell tracking [30]. Free [^{64}Cu]$CuCl_2$ can also been used as a valuable radiopharmaceutical for quantifying physiological biodistribution of Cu in associated disorders including Wilson's and Menkes diseases in preclinical studies [29, 31], Alzheimer's disease [32, 33], and cancer PET imaging (e.g., prostate cancer) [34]. Also, preclinical studies have shown the diagnostic efficiency of [^{64}Cu]$CuCl_2$ in a glioblastoma xenograft model [35]. Suitable visualization of the tumor by [^{64}Cu]$CuCl_2$ can provide a theory that supports the non-dependency of ^{64}Cu complexes on ligands for tumor accumulations [35]. The following passages will discuss notable applications of ^{64}Cu radiopharmaceuticals in accomplished clinical trials with the aim of clarifying new PET tracers' roles in nuclear medicine.

1.2 Imaging tumor hypoxia

In circumstances under which cells are deprived of oxygen, hypoxia will occur and resistance to radiotherapy or chemotherapy and risk of invasion and metastases increases [11, 36, 37]. Hypoxia is a common condition in 50–60% of locally advanced solid tumors [11]. In addition to variable levels in different tumors, heterogeneity in a particular tumor tissue also can affect the reliable estimation of hypoxia [38]. Given a specific physiological state in hypoxia cells, they can be diagnosed with medical imaging modalities [39]. As a result, there are various PET tracers, which specifically detect hypoxia in humans [40–42]. In a series of *ex-vivo* studies, Fujibayashi et al. initially identified the critical role of the lipophilic radioactive copper (II) complex of the N_2S_2 ligand termed [^{62}Cu]Cu-ATSM, specifically in relation to selective accumulation in hypoxia cells [43, 44]. Later, *in-vivo* studies demonstrated further that copper radiolabeled ATSMs have high specificity and selectivity as tracers for the detection of tumor hypoxia [45–49]. Despite the fact that the exact localization mechanism of Cu-ATSM is still not fully understood, theoretical evaluations suggest that Cu-ATSM can passively diffuse through cell membranes due to its high permeability. Moreover, due to the low redox potential of the tracer, it can be trapped constantly following the reduction process in hypoxic cells [14]. This reduction can only occur in hypoxic cells given that the abnormally reduced state of their mitochondria is not common in normoxic cells [43].

In a comparison study by Lewis et al., [^{64}Cu]Cu-ATSM, [^{64}Cu]Cu-PTSM, and [^{18}F]F-MISO were identified as the most promising tumor hypoxia radiopharmaceuticals while also showing that the former ([^{64}Cu]Cu-ATSM), exhibits heterogeneous oxygen concentration-dependent accumulation in different cells compared to the more stable uptake of the [^{64}Cu]Cu-PTSM and [^{18}F]F-MISO [50]. Also, [^{64}Cu]Cu-ATSM presented faster clearance from normal tissues compared to the other tumor hypoxia tracers [51]. All in all, previous data show that PET/CT utilizing [^{64}Cu]Cu-ATSM is a reliable and non-invasive imaging method that can accurately map hypoxic areas [52, 53]. In a clinical study of 10 cervical cancer patients, results showed that the signal-to-noise ratio was superior for [^{64}Cu]Cu-ATSM was superior to [^{60}Cu]Cu-ATSM. Consequently, [^{64}Cu]Cu-ATSM has been proposed as a safe radiopharmaceutical that can be used to achieve high-quality imaging in tumor hypoxia cases [54]. Moreover, these data also showed that imaging reproducibility is feasible for up to 9 days. Accordingly, the authors concluded that [^{64}Cu]Cu-ATSM is an ideal radiotracer for chronic tumor hypoxia rather than as an acute condition [55].

Furthermore, in a case report on a glioblastoma multiforme (GBM) patient, the authors observed accumulation of [^{64}Cu]Cu-ATSM from early acquisition to late acquisition in hypoxia sites as well as high correlation between ^{64}Cu-ATSM PET/CT results and HIF-1α expression as a hypoxia marker [56]. Feasibility of ^{64}Cu-ATSM PET/CT in both cervical cancer and lung cancer has also been previously demonstrated [57–59], while in a comparative clinical study in 11 patients with head and neck cancer treated with chemoradiotherapy, the efficacy of [^{64}Cu]Cu-ATSM and [^{18}F]FDG was evaluated [60]. According to the findings of [^{64}Cu]Cu-ATSM in seven patients, nodal metastases were detected and 22 cancer foci were identified in total calculated amounts for sensitivity and specificity of [^{64}Cu]Cu-ATSM based on evaluated SUVmax were 100 and 50% and the same estimation considering the volume were 100 and 33%, respectively [60]. In conventional theories accumulation mechanism of [^{64}Cu]Cu-ATSM was interpreted based on ^{64}Cu(II) oxidation state [43, 61]. It was proposed that ^{64}Cu(II) be reduced to ^{64}Cu(I) by NADH/NADPH under the hypoxia circumstances. According to the lower stability of ^{64}Cu(I) compared to ^{64}Cu(II) dissociation of the [^{64}Cu]Cu-ATSM results in H2-ATSM and free Cu ions [50]. However, the exact reduction process is under debate until now. Colombié et al. reported that the functional mechanism of [^{64}Cu(II)]-Cu-ATSM is related to redox potential and formation of reactive oxygen species which can appear under the hypoxia cellular condition [53]. Further studies suggest that the accumulation of [^{64}Cu(II)]-Cu-ATSM is not mediated depending on the oxygen pressure of the tumors [62]. In sum, these results show a comparable efficacy between [^{64}Cu] Cu-ATSM and [^{18}F]FDG PET/CT in the estimation of biological tumor volume (BTV), while clarifying that [^{64}Cu]Cu-ATSM has higher sensitivity and lower specificity in predicting neoadjuvant chemoradiotherapy responses [60].

1.3 Tumor targeting by radiolabeled antibodies

1.3.1 [^{64}Cu]Cu-trastuzumab

Epidermal growth factor receptor (ErbB) is composed of four closely related members including ErbB-1 (HER1 or epidermal growth factor receptor, EGFR), ErbB-2 (HER2), ErbB-3 (HER3), and ErbB-4 (HER4). HER1, HER3, and HER4 bind to approximately a dozen of different ligands while HER2 has no specific ligand [63, 64]. Previously, it has been demonstrated that HER2 is activated through dimerization with other HER derivatives. This complex will subsequently activate intracellular signaling pathways of MAPK (mitogen-activated protein kinase) and PI3K (phosphoinositide 3-kinase) [65]. These pathways are responsible for tumor growth, invasion, migration, and survival while gene coding associated with breast cancer can amplify 15–20% of them [66, 67]. Gene amplification or protein overexpression are notable criteria for the candidacy of breast cancer patients from primary to metastatic stages for HER2-directed therapy [63]. Trastuzumab is confirmed as the first-line of a therapeutic plan for HER2-positive in advanced breast cancer [68]. Trastuzumab is a humanized antibody that binds to the extracellular domain of HER2 and inhibits the proliferation progress [69]. It was demonstrated as a remarkable point that [^{64}Cu]Cu-trastuzumab can be used for pretreatment assessment of breast cancer. Since measurements of [^{64}Cu]Cu-trastuzumab uptake in lesions is a very promising criterion of patient selection for treatment procedures [63]. In a clinical trial performed of five HER2-positive breast cancer patients, results indicated that [^{64}Cu]Cu-trastuzumab PET/CT scan is a safe and feasible for non-invasive and serial detection of HER2 status in metastatic brain tumors [70]. Based on clinical trials, [^{64}Cu]Cu-trastuzumab can be efficient for the diagnosis of metastases related to other malignancies [71]. For instance, radiolabeled trastuzumab can be mentioned as a standard tracer for HER2-positive gastric or gastro-esophageal junction cancer patients [72]. Moreover, a recent clinical trial compared [^{64}Cu]Cu-NOTA-trastuzumab in a HER2-positive primary gastric cancer patient with liver metastases, to [^{18}F]FDG [73] with results showing comparable outcomes. Specifically, six liver metastases >1 cm were identified by both detection radiopharmaceuticals. Two metastases <0.5 cm were detected only with [^{18}F]FDG and were not easily identified with [^{64}Cu]Cu-NOTA-trastuzumab [73]. However, SUVmax of [^{64}Cu]Cu-NOTA-trastuzumab in the primary lesion was estimated 28.6 ± 0.50 versus 13.5 ± 0.30 for [^{18}F]FDG [73]. Based on comparable clinical results between [^{18}F]FDG and [^{64}Cu]Cu-trastuzumab attained by these data, it can be argued that further clinical evaluations of [^{64}Cu]Cu-trastuzumab are needed.

1.3.2 [^{64}Cu]Cu-rituximab

Rituximab (RTX) is a chimeric human/murine mAb that targets CD20 positive B-cell malignancies and has been used for immunotherapy of patients with non-Hodgkin's lymphoma (NHL) [74, 75]. Radiolabeling of RTX with (β^-/β^+) emitters could augment the antibodies' theranostic activity. In this regard, ^{64}Cu-labeled RTX ([^{64}Cu]Cu-DOTA-rituximab) as a PET imaging agent could be used to track the progress of NHL treatment [75]. The ongoing pre-clinical trial using [^{64}Cu]Cu-DOTA-rituximab PET/CT was established to determine the tracers' pharmacokinetics, biodistribution, stability, uptake, and radiation dosimetry in CD20-positive B-cell NHL patients compared to the [^{18}F]FDG PET/CT [76]. Following this study, Natarjan et al. reported validated production of [^{64}Cu]Cu-rituximab under good manufacturing practices (GMP) in order to clinical indication for the diagnosis of CD20 positive B-cell non-Hodgkin lymphoma [75]. Finally based on strong evidences efficacy of [^{64}Cu]Cu-rituximab in detecting of B-cells in a murine model of MS was confirmed [77]. This achievement can be very hopeful in detection or even early diagnosis of MS in patients who respond to anti-B-cell therapies.

1.4 Tumor targeting by radiolabeled somatostatin derivatives: [^{64}Cu]Cu-DOTA-TATE, and [^{64}Cu]Cu-DOTA-TOC

Somatostatin receptors (SSTR) have been reported as qualified targets for the evaluation of neuroendocrine tumors (NETs) [78]. After [^{68}Ga]Ga-DOTA-TATE, which was introduced as a gold standard for diagnosis purposes of NETs, it was hypothesized that ^{64}Cu would be superior for radiolabeling of somatostatin derivatives [78]. The physical properties of ^{64}Cu compared to ^{68}Ga, including longer half-life (12.7 h versus 67.7 min for ^{68}Ga), and shorter positron range (1 mm versus 4 mm), makes ^{64}Cu more accessible radionuclide with higher spatial resolution for clinical studies [79]. Various comparative studies have been performed to clarify the emphasis of radiolabeled somatostatin derivatives with ^{64}Cu. In a clinical trial study of 59 NET patients carried out by Johnbeck and colleagues, the authors compared diagnostic results derived from [^{68}Ga]Ga-DOTA-TOC and [^{64}Cu]Cu-DOTA-TATE PET/CT radiopharmaceuticals [78]. Results showed that 701 lesions were concordantly recognized with both radiopharmaceuticals. However, in detection of 68 lesions, there were no correlation between the [^{68}Ga]Ga-DOTA-TOC and [^{64}Cu]Cu-DOTA-TATE. Forty-two lesions were detected only by [^{64}Cu]Cu-DOTA-TATE, of which 33 were found to be true positives. Moreover, only 26 lesions were found with [^{68}Ga]Ga-DOTA-TOC, of which seven were true positive [78]. These results demonstrated that [^{64}Cu]Cu-DOTA-TATE exhibits higher specificity and sensitivity compared to [^{68}Ga]Ga-DOTA-TOC [78].

Further studies have confirmed that [^{64}Cu]Cu-DOTA-TATE's role as a safe imaging protocol in providing of accurate and high-quality images for diagnosis, treatment, and follow-up of NETs [80–83]. In accomplished comparative clinical studies for [^{64}Cu]Cu-DOTA-TATE, [^{99m}Tc]Tc-HYNIC-octreotide, and [^{111}In]In-DTPA-OC, superiority of [^{64}Cu]Cu-DOTA-TATE in the diagnosis of NETs was demonstrated [82, 84]. [^{64}Cu]Cu-DOTA-TATE is the most appropriate choice for the diagnosis of NETs due to robust manufacturing with no need for regional generators, and a longer half-life allowing a wide geographical range for commercial distribution. This drug was approved in September 2020 by FDA and is now commercially available in the USA. **Figures 1–3** display detection rate of [^{64}Cu]Cu-DOTA-TATE in NETs. In a clinical trial [^{64}Cu]Cu-MeCOSar-Tyr^{3}-octreotate ([^{64}Cu]Cu-SARTATE) was applied in [^{68}Ga]Ga-DOTA-TATE positive NET patients [85]. A significant advantage of this radiopharmaceutical compared to [^{68}Ga]Ga-DOTA-TATE is the higher stability of sarcophagine (Sar) linker versus DOTA. The concluded results showed comparable diagnosis visualization in 9 of 10 patients in 1 h imaging. In one patient a liver lesion was missed by [^{64}Cu]Cu-SARTATE. However, the imaging obtained in 24 h, demonstrated the diagnostic superiority of [^{64}Cu]Cu-SARTATE compared to [^{68}Ga]Ga-DOTA-TATE [85].

Several somatostatins analogs radiolabeled with SPECT and PET radionuclides have been evaluated in clinical trials to ascertain a possible gold standard for the diagnosis and treatment of NETs [86]. To date, 68Ga radiolabeled somatostatin derivatives including DOTA-TOC, DOTA-TATE, and DOTA-NOC (**Figure 4**) have shown promising results as diagnostic radiopharmaceuticals for NETs [78]. Recently, it was also demonstrated that 64Cu radiolabeled somatostatin analogs have advantages compared to former radiopharmaceuticals, some of which are discussed previously.

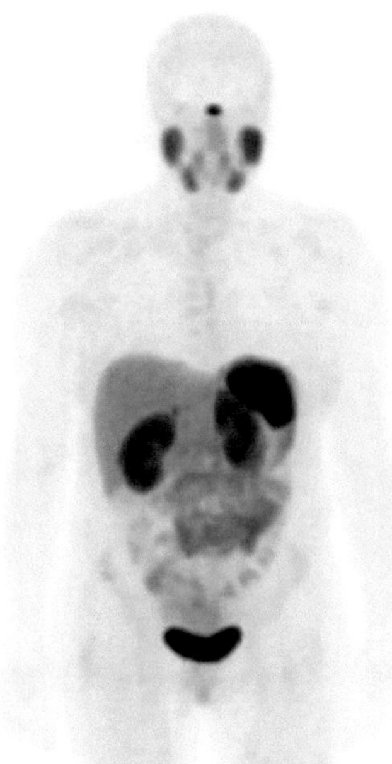

Figure 1.
Physiologic uptake is seen in the pituitary, salivary, and lacrimal glands, liver, spleen, GI tract, adrenals, kidneys, and urinary bladder. Mild & diffuse bone marrow uptake or focal activity in the pancreas might occur as normal physiologic variants (e.g., uncinate process of the pancreas). (Courtesy of Courtesy Ebrahim Delpassand, MD RadioMedix, Inc. Houston, TX, USA).

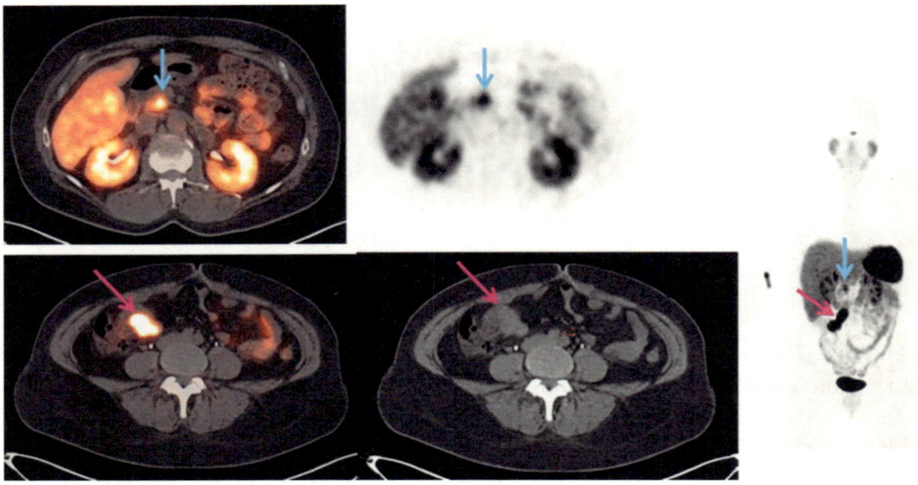

Figure 2.
53-year-old female with newly diagnosed neuroendocrine tumor in the terminal ileum. The red arrow points to the primary tumor. The blue arrow points to the uncinate process uptake, which is a normal physiological variant. (Courtesy Ebrahim Delpassand, MD, RadioMedix, Inc. Houston, TX, USA).

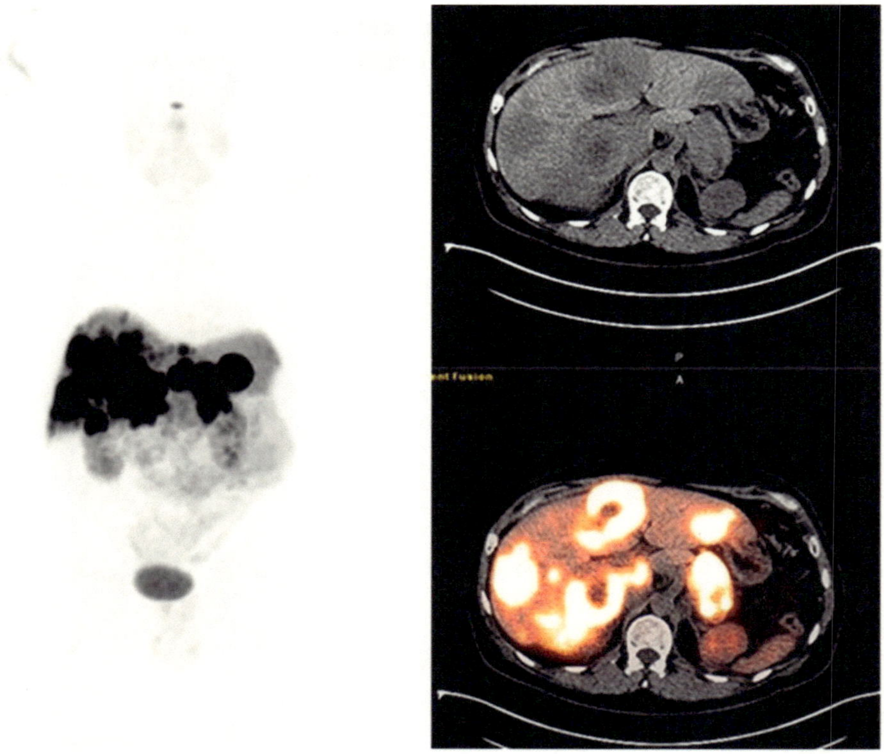

Figure 3.
49-year-old male with pancreatic neuroendocrine tumor. On the fused [^{64}Cu]Cu-DOTA-TATE PET/CT images a [^{64}Cu]Cu-DOTA-TATE avid lesion is noted in the pancreatic tail. Also, multiple hypodense [^{64}Cu]Cu-DOTA-TATE avid lesions are noted in both liver lobes suggesting metastatic involvement. (Courtesy Courtesy Ebrahim Delpassand, MD RadioMedix, Inc. Houston, TX, USA).

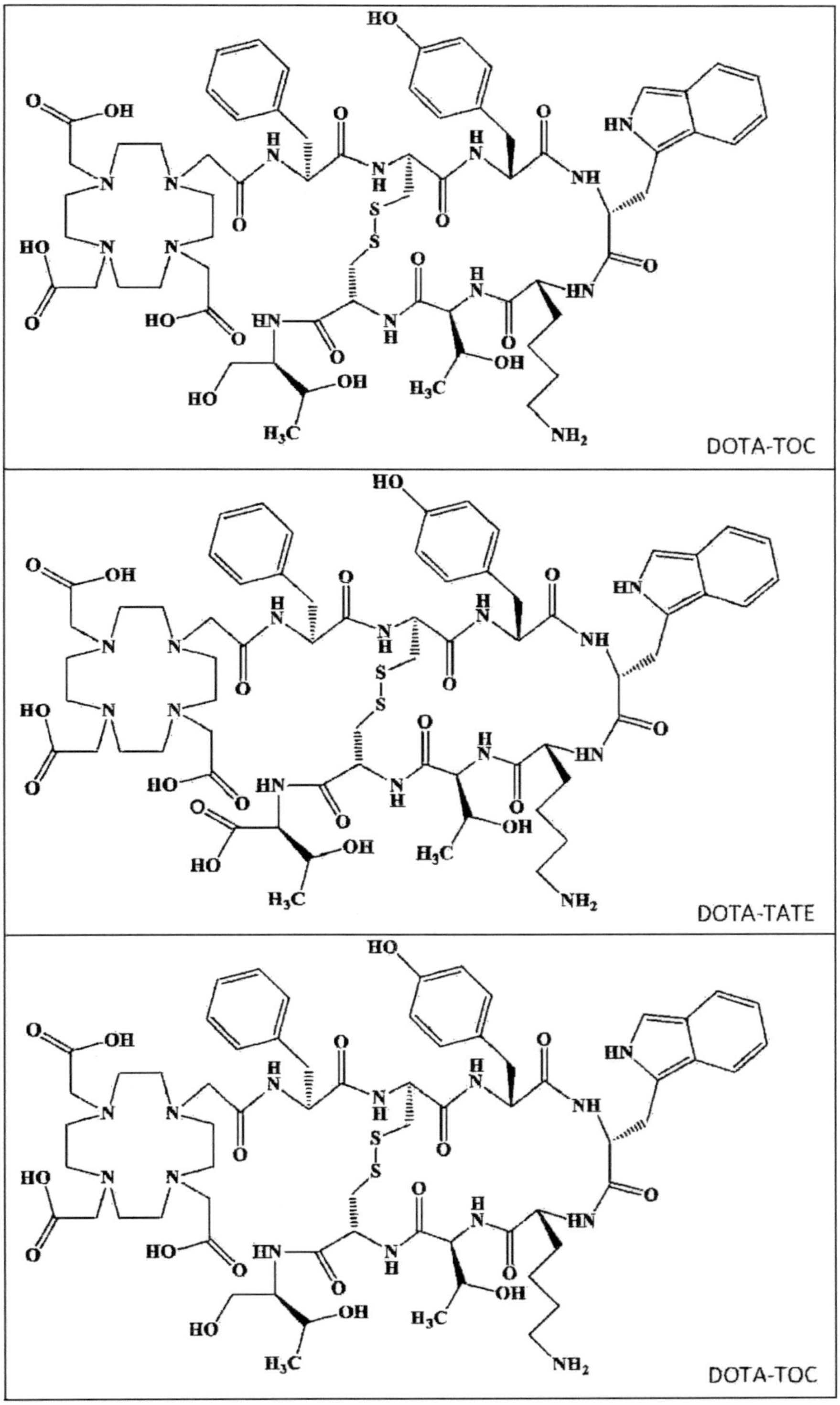

Figure 4.
Chemical structures of DOTA-TOC (top), DOTA-TATE (middle), and DOTA-NOC (bottom).

In a retrospective study, 33 patients with NETs who had surgically removed primary lesions, underwent [^{64}Cu]Cu-DOTA-TOC PET/CT scan [87]. Five patients exhibited no detectable pathological lesion in PET/CT scan, while eight showed enhanced uptake at the skull base, and 20 presented at least one pathological lesion [87]. Based on this clinical trial, it was concluded that [64Cu]Cu-DOTA-TOC PET/CT scan can differentiate NET lesions with a feature of high target-to-background contrast [87]. Interestingly, these findings also correlated with [177Lu]Lu-DOTA-TATE results obtained from a follow-up assessment in another patient's group [87]. Further studies on larger populations are needed to identify the most appropriate somatostatin derivative for NETs diagnosis in radiolabeling with 64Cu. As an example, (**Figure 5**) displays the detection rate of [^{64}Cu]Cu-DOTA-TOC in NET of the bladder.

1.5 Tumor targeting by radiolabeled PSMA ligands

1.5.1 [^{64}Cu]Cu-PSMA-617

Previous studies have been demonstrated that prostate-specific membrane antigen (PSMA) is over expressed in prostate cancer (PCa) [88], suggesting that PSMA can be used as a potent tumor marker for PCa, as well as a vital target for imaging and therapy [88]. Among the recognized radiolabeled PSMA inhibitors, it has been shown that [^{68}Ga]Ga-PSMA-11 is highly effective as a PET tracer for the detection of PCa [88]. Furthermore, PSMA can also be radiolabeled with ^{64}Cu, offering a longer half-life and higher spatial resolution [89]. In a comparative clinical trial, the biodistribution of [^{64}Cu]Cu-PSMA-617 and [^{68}Ga]Ga-PSMA-11 were assessed in PCa patients [89]. Diagnostic results showed that both radiopharmaceuticals show similar biodistribution, except the excretion route, in which [^{64}Cu]Cu-PSMA-617 excreting takes place through the gastrointestinal tract rather than the renal excretion of [^{68}Ga] Ga-PSMA-11 [89]. The low metabolic rate of PCa cells leads to negligible uptake of [^{18}F]FDG in PCa. [^{18}F]FDG accumulates based on glucose consumption and as a consequence of the mentioned fact unacceptable specificity of [^{18}F]FDG for the detection of PCa is raised [90–92]. However, it has also been demonstrated that [^{18}F] FDG is useful for selected PCa patients with hormone-resistant poorly differentiated cell types [93–95].

Choline is an essential precursor for phospholipid synthesis of membranes in normal cells and based on the proliferation rate, uptake of choline increases mainly in cancerous cells [96, 97]. [^{18}F]F-choline ([^{18}F]FCH) PET/CT has been used for the detection of PCa widely during the last decade and optimistic results have been achieved [90]. It assessed that [^{18}F]FCH PET/CT is useful for detection of local and distant nodal recurrence and bone metastases [90, 98–100]. In another cohort study, the efficacy of [^{64}Cu]Cu-PSMA-617 and [^{18}F]FCH PET/CT was compared [101]. This study, conducted on 43 patients, assessed restaging after biochemical recurrence [101]. In terms of detection rate, results indicated no statistically significant differences. However, [^{64}Cu]Cu-PSMA-617 showed better performance with overall positivity at 74.4% compared to 44.2% for [^{18}F]FCH [101]. This retrospective study demonstrated that [^{64}Cu]Cu-PSMA-617 is promising in the prediction and assessment of recurrent sites relative to other PET tracers [101].

In another clinical trial performed by Grubmuller et al., it was shown that [^{64}Cu] Cu-PSMA-617 has high potential as a PET tracer in detection of recurrent cases or progressive local lesions in primary staging of PCa patients [102]. In comparison to [^{68}Ga]

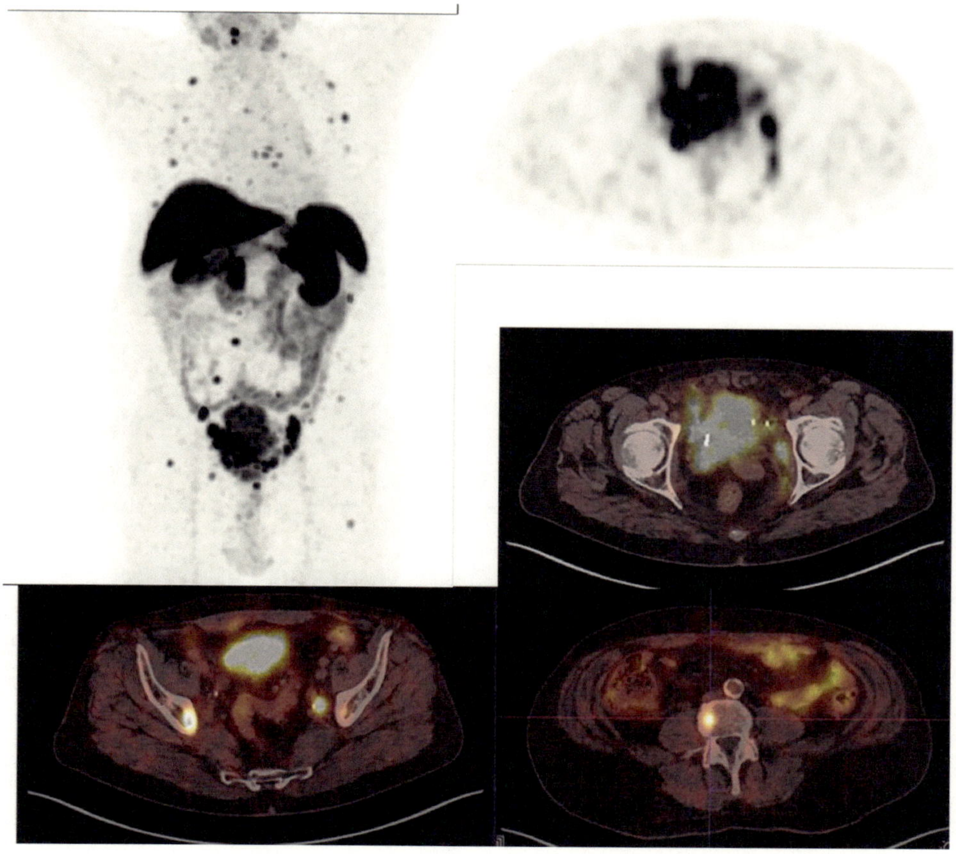

Figure 5.
68-year-old male patient with a neuroendocrine tumor of the bladder (G3) with multiple pelvic LN and bone metastases. Additionally, we see the primary tumor in the bladder with infiltration into the surrounding tissue. [^{64}Cu]Cu-DOTA-TOC (179 MBq) PET/CT. (Courtesy of Clinic Ottakring, Institute of Nuclear Medicine with PET-Center, Vienna, Austria).

Ga-PSMA-11, higher image quality resulting from higher image contrast and superior uptake for [^{64}Cu]Cu-PSMA-617 was shown, suggests the latter as an appropriate radiopharmaceutical compared to conventional PCa radiotracers [102]. Subsequently, [^{64}Cu]$CuCl_2$ has also been reported as an applicable diagnostic tracer for PCa [34, 103]. Cu is an essential requirement for normal cells in signaling transduction pathways of proliferation processes [104]. So increased uptake of Cu in aggressive uncontrolled cancerous prostate cells with a high proliferation rate would be inevitable [103]. In a previous study 50 patients with biochemical relapse PCa after surgery or external beam radiation therapy went through [^{64}Cu]$CuCl_2$ and [^{18}F]F-choline PET/CT scans [34], results indicated that biodistribution of [^{64}Cu]$CuCl_2$ is more appropriate for exploring the prostate and pelvic bed. Finally, it was shown that in patients with relapsed PCa and low levels of PSA, [^{64}Cu]$CuCl_2$ has a higher detection rate compared to [^{18}F]F-choline [34]. In sum, it can be argued that [^{64}Cu]$CuCl_2$ is a suitable tracer for the primary staging of PCa and regional lymph nodes [103]. However, based on high diagnostic accuracy, [^{64}Cu]Cu-PSMA-617 has been suggested in both primary staging in patients with progressive local disease and recurrent cases [102, 105, 106].

Pharmaceutical	Dose (MBq)	Average effective dose (mSv/MBq)	Study type	Organs with highest absorbed dose (mGy/MBq)	Ref.
[^{64}Cu]Cu-DOTA-trastuzumab	115–136	0.036 ± 0.009 (mean: 4.5 mSv)	Patient	Heart: 0.340	[71]
				Liver: 0.237	
				Spleen: 0.142	
[^{64}Cu]Cu-NOTA-trastuzumab	3.7	—	Animal/ Monte Carlo simulation	Heart: 0.048	[107]
				Liver: 0.079	
				Spleen: 0.047	
[^{64}Cu] Cu-PSMA-617	18.7[*] 119–160[#]	0.0292	Animal/ patient	Gallbladder wall: 2.04	[108]
				Liver: 0.014	
				Kidney: 0.009	
[^{64}Cu] Cu-DOTA-TATE	193–232	0.0315	Patient	Pituitary gland: 0.19	[109]
				Liver: 0.16	
				Kidneys: 0.14	
[^{64}Cu]Cu-DOTA-pembrolizumab	7.4	0.004	Animal[a]	Liver: 0.032	[110]
				Red marrow: 0.018	
				Lungs: 0.010	
[^{64}Cu]Cu-TETA-OC	107–130[#]	0.013	Animal/ patient	Bladder wall: 0.25	[111]
				Liver: 0.092	
				Kidneys: 0.078	
[^{64}Cu] Cu-DOTA-AE105	197–213	0.0276	Human	Liver: 0.175	[112]
				Kidney: 0.0562	
[^{64}Cu]Cu-DOTA-alendronate	37–74	0.0418	Animal[b]	LLI wall: 0.159	[113]
				ULI wall: 0.113	
				Kidneys: 0.108	
[^{64}Cu]Cu-Cl_2	4.0 MBq/ kg	0.051 (m)	Human	Liver: 0.310 (m)	[114]
				Liver: 0.421 (f)	
		0.061 (f)		LLI wall: 0.153 (m)	
				LLI wall: 0.161 (f)	
[$^{60/61/62/64}$Cu] Cu-ATSM	480[1]	0.011[1]	Animal/ patients[c]	Liver: 0.064[1]	[115]
		0.029[2]		Liver: 0.275[2]	
		0.003[3]		Liver: 0.017[3]	
		0.036[4]		Liver: 0.390[4]	
[^{64}Cu] Cu-SARTATE	192	0.0454	Human	Spleen: 0.361	[85]
				Kidneys: 0.202	
				Adernals: 0.169	

DOI: http://dx.doi.org/10.5772/intechopen.1003993

Pharmaceutical	Dose (MBq)	Average effective dose (mSv/MBq)	Study type	Organs with highest absorbed dose (mGy/MBq)	Ref.
$[^{64}Cu]$Cu-DOTA-Rituximab	7.4	0.024	Animal[b]	Spleen: 0.098	[76]
				Liver: 0.051	
				Osteogenic cells: 0.042	

LLI wall: lower large intestine wall.
ULI wall: upper large intestine wall.
m: men.
f: women.
[*]mice.
[#]patient.
[1]copper-60.
[2]copper-61.
[3]copper-62.
[4]copper-64.
[a]based on ex-vivo biodistribution and PET/CT images.
[b]estimation for humans.
[c]dose estimation for human based on copper-60.

Table 3.
Injected dose level, estimated absorbed doses, and organs at risk in $[^{64}Cu]$Cu-radiopharmaceuticals.

2. Pre-clinical and clinical dosimetry results of ^{64}Cu-radiopharmaceuticals

Table 3 shows the results of the injected dose level and the estimated absorbed doses and organs at risk in ^{64}Cu radiopharmaceuticals. Based on previous studies on ^{64}Cu-radiopharmaceuticals, injected dose levels for patients were between 105 and 192 MBq which is about half of $[^{18}F]$FDG dose and provided acceptable image quality. The calculated effective absorbed dose for the total body with ^{64}Cu-radiopharmaceuticals in human studies or in animal studies indicated a range of 0.01–0.06 mSv/MBq. In the case of radiation potential hazards, these ranges are within an acceptable level and lower than other similar radiopharmaceuticals.

3. Conclusion

The number of developing ^{64}Cu labeled radiopharmaceuticals is growing. The most considerable characteristics of ^{64}Cu include a longer half-life and superior image quality, resulting in high image contrasts, robust centralized manufacturing, and wider geographical range of distribution and ease of use by the end user. These characteristics have led to the introduction of novel and promising ^{64}Cu radiopharmaceuticals in both pre-clinical and clinical trials. $[^{64}Cu]$Cu- DOTATATE (Detectnet™) is the first ^{64}Cu labeled radiopharmaceutical approved by the FDA and is commercially available in the USA. ^{64}Cu/^{67}Cu pair has great and true theranostic applications. Impressive numbers of clinical trials using ^{64}Cu labeled compounds suggest that the menu of approved radiopharmaceuticals in this field will increase in the near future.

Abbreviations

ATSM:	diacetyl-bis(N4-methylthiosemicarbazone)
BTV:	biological tumor volume
CD20:	cluster of differentiate 20
CT:	computed tomography
Cu:	copper
DOTA:	2,2′,2”,2”'-(1,4,7,10-tetraazacyclododecane-1,4,7,10-tetrayl)tetraacetic acid
FCH:	fluorocholine
FDG:	fludeoxyglucose
FDA:	food and drug administration
Ga:	gallium
GBM:	glioblastoma multiform
GI:	gastro intestinal
HER:	human epidermal growth factor receptor
MAb:	monoclonal antibody
MAPK:	mitogen-activated protein kinases
MBq:	mega becquerel
MISO:	misonidazole
NADH:	nicotinamide adenine dinucleotide (NAD) + hydrogen (H)
NADPH:	nicotinamide adenine dinucleotide phosphate
NET:	neuroendocrine tumors
NHL:	non-Hodgkin lymphoma
NOC:	[Nal3]-octreotide
NOTA:	2,2′-(7-(2-((2,5-dioxopyrrolidin-1-yl)oxy)-2-oxoethyl)-1,4,7-triazonane-1,4-diyl)diacetic acid
PCa:	prostate cancer
PET:	positron emission tomography
PTSM:	pyruvaldehyde-bis(N4-methylthiosemicarbazone)
PSA:	prostate specific antigen
PSMA:	prostate specific membrane antigen
RTX:	Rituximab
SAR:	sarcophagine
SPECT:	single-photon emission computed tomography
SSTR:	somatostatin receptor
TATE:	[Tyr3]-octreotate
TOC:	[Tyr3]-octreotide

Author details

Nasim Vahidfar[1], Mohsen Bakhshi Kashi[1], Saeed Afshar[1], Peyman Sheikhzadeh[1], Saeed Farzanefar[1], Yalda Salehi[1], Ebrahim Delpasand[2,3], Eóin N. Molloy[4,5], Siroos Mirzaei[6], Hojjat Ahmadzadehfar[7] and Elisabeth Eppard[4]*

1 Department of Nuclear Medicine, Vali-Asr Hospital, Tehran University of Medical Sciences, Tehran, Iran

2 RadioMedix, Inc., Houston, TX, USA

3 Excel Diagnostics and Nuclear Oncology Center, Houston, TX, USA

4 University Clinic for Radiology and Nuclear Medicine, Faculty of Medicine, Otto von Guericke University (OvGU), Magdeburg, Germany

5 Multimodal Neuroimaging Lab, German Centre for Neurodegenerative Diseases, Magdeburg, Germany

6 Clinic Ottakring, Institute of Nuclear Medicine with PET-Center, Vienna, Austria

7 Department of Nuclear Medicine, Klinikum Westfalen, Dortmund, Germany

*Address all correspondence to: elisabeth.eppard@med.ovgu.de

References

[1] Boschi A, Martini P, Janevik-Ivanovska E, Duatti A. The emerging role of copper-64 radiopharmaceuticals as cancer theranostics. Drug Discovery Today. 2018;**23**:1489-1501

[2] Oyen W, Bodei L, Giammarile F, Maecke H, Tennvall J, Luster M, et al. Targeted therapy in nuclear medicine—Current status and future prospects. Annals of Oncology. 2007;**18**:1782-1792

[3] Stéen EJL, Edem PE, Nørregaard K, Jørgensen JT, Shalgunov V, Kjaer A, et al. Pretargeting in nuclear imaging and radionuclide therapy: Improving efficacy of theranostics and nanomedicines. Biomaterials. 2018;**179**:209-245

[4] Ma MT, Donnelly PS. Peptide targeted copper-64 radiopharmaceuticals. Current Topics in Medicinal Chemistry. 2011;**11**:500-520

[5] Jones T, Townsend DW. History and future technical innovation in positron emission tomography. Journal of Medical Imaging. 2017;**4**:011013

[6] Duclos V, Iep A, Gomez L, Goldfarb L, Besson FL. PET molecular imaging: A holistic review of current practice and emerging perspectives for diagnosis, therapeutic evaluation and prognosis in clinical oncology. International Journal of Molecular Sciences. 2021;**22**:4159

[7] Lebech A-M, Gaardsting A, Loft A, Graff J, Markova E, Bertelsen AK, et al. Whole-body 18F-FDG PET/CT is superior to CT as first-line diagnostic imaging in patients referred with serious nonspecific symptoms or signs of cancer: A randomized prospective study of 200 patients. Journal of Nuclear Medicine. 2017;**58**:1058-1064

[8] International BR. Retracted: The copper radioisotopes: A systematic review with special interest to 64Cu. BioMed Research International. 2018;**2018**:1. Article ID 3860745. DOI: 10.1155/2018/3860745

[9] Williams HA, Robinson S, Julyan P, Zweit J, Hastings D. A comparison of PET imaging characteristics of various copper radioisotopes. European Journal of Nuclear Medicine and Molecular Imaging. 2005;**32**:1473-1480

[10] Kodama H, Fujisawa C. Copper metabolism and inherited coppertransport disorders: Molecular mechanisms, screening, and treatment. Metallomics. 2009;**1**:42-52

[11] Hao G, Singh AN, Oz OK, Sun X. Recent advances in copper radiopharmaceuticals. Current Radiopharmaceuticals. 2011;**4**:109-121

[12] Tapiero H, Townsend DÁ, Tew K. Trace elements in human physiology and pathology. Copper. Biomedicine & Pharmacotherapy. 2003;**57**:386-398

[13] Gutfilen B, Souza SA, Valentini G. Copper-64: A real theranostic agent. Drug Design, Development and Therapy. 2018;**12**:3235

[14] Zhou Y, Li J, Xu X, Zhao M, Zhang B, Deng S, et al. 64Cu-based radiopharmaceuticals in molecular imaging. Technology in Cancer Research & Treatment. 2019;**18**:1533033819830758

[15] Bhargava KK, Gupta RK, Nichols KJ, Palestro CJ. In vitro human leukocyte labeling with 64Cu: An intraindividual comparison with 111In-oxine and 18F-FDG. Nuclear Medicine and Biology. 2009;**36**:545-549

[16] Niccoli Asabella A, Cascini GL, Altini C, Paparella D, Notaristefano A, Rubini G. The copper radioisotopes: A systematic review with special interest to 64Cu. BioMed Research International. 7 May 2014;**2014**:786463. DOI: 10.1155/2014/786463

[17] Lewis JS, Herrero P, Sharp TL, Engelbach JA, Fujibayashi Y, Laforest R, et al. Delineation of hypoxia in canine myocardium using PET and copper (II)-diacetyl-bis(N4-methylthiosemicarbazone). Journal of Nuclear Medicine. 2002;**43**:1557-1569

[18] Holland JP, Ferdani R, Anderson CJ, Lewis JS. Copper-64 radiopharmaceuticals for oncologic imaging. PET Clinics. 2009;**4**:49-67

[19] Jauregui-Osoro M, De Robertis S, Halsted P, Gould S-M, Yu Z, Paul RL, et al. Production of copper-64 using a hospital cyclotron: Targetry, purification and quality analysis. Nuclear Medicine Communications. 2021;**42**:1024

[20] Jødal L, Le Loirec C, Champion C. Positron range in PET imaging: Non-conventional isotopes. Physics in Medicine & Biology. 2014;**59**:7419

[21] Palmer MR, Zhu X, Parker JA. Modeling and simulation of positron range effects for high resolution PET imaging. IEEE Transactions on Nuclear Science. 2005;**52**:1391-1395

[22] Dearling JL, Lewis JS, Mullen GE, Welch MJ, Blower PJ. Copper bis (thiosemicarbazone) complexes as hypoxia imaging agents: Structure-activity relationships. JBIC Journal of Biological Inorganic Chemistry. 2002;**7**:249-259

[23] Handley MG, Medina RA, Mariotti E, Kenny GD, Shaw KP, Yan R, et al. Cardiac hypoxia imaging: Second-generation analogues of 64Cu-ATSM. Journal of Nuclear Medicine. 2014;**55**:488-494

[24] Fleming IN, Manavaki R, Blower PJ, West C, Williams KJ, Harris AL, et al. Imaging tumour hypoxia with positron emission tomography. British Journal of Cancer. 2015;**112**:238-250

[25] Wallhaus TR, Lacy J, Stewart R, Bianco J, Green MA, Nayak N, et al. Copper-62-pyruvaldehyde bis (N4-methyl-thiosemicarbazone) PET imaging in the detection of coronary artery disease in humans. Journal of Nuclear Cardiology. 2001;**8**:67-74

[26] Peng F, Lutsenko S, Sun X, Muzik O. Imaging copper metabolism imbalance in Atp7b−/− knockout mouse model of Wilson's disease with PET-CT and orally administered 64 CuCl 2. Molecular Imaging and Biology. 2012;**14**:600-607

[27] Andreozzi EM, Torres JB, Sunassee K, Dunn J, Walker-Samuel S, Szanda I, et al. Studies of copper trafficking in a mouse model of Alzheimer's disease by positron emission tomography: Comparison of 64Cu acetate and 64CuGTSM. Metallomics. 2017;**9**:1622-1633

[28] Bartnicka JJ, Blower PJ. Insights into trace metal metabolism in health and disease from PET:"PET Metallomics". Journal of Nuclear Medicine. 2018;**59**:1355-1359

[29] Torres JB, Andreozzi EM, Dunn JT, Siddique M, Szanda I, Howlett DR, et al. PET imaging of copper trafficking in a mouse model of Alzheimer disease. Journal of Nuclear Medicine. 2016;**57**:109-114

[30] Griessinger CM, Kehlbach R, Bukala D, Wiehr S, Bantleon R, Cay F, et al. In vivo tracking of Th1 cells by

PET reveals quantitative and temporal distribution and specific homing in lymphatic tissue. Journal of Nuclear Medicine. 2014;**55**:301-307

[31] Nomura S, Nozaki S, Hamazaki T, Takeda T, Ninomiya E, Kudo S, et al. PET imaging analysis with 64Cu in disulfiram treatment for aberrant copper biodistribution in Menkes disease mouse model. Journal of Nuclear Medicine. 2014;**55**:845-851

[32] Fodero-Tavoletti MT, Villemagne VL, Paterson BM, White AR, Li Q-X, Camakaris J, et al. Bis (thiosemicarbazonato) Cu-64 complexes for positron emission tomography imaging of Alzheimer's disease. Journal of Alzheimer's Disease. 2010;**20**:49-55

[33] Hickey JL, Lim S, Hayne DJ, Paterson BM, White JM, Villemagne VL, et al. Diagnostic imaging agents for Alzheimer's disease: Copper radiopharmaceuticals that target Aβ plaques. Journal of the American Chemical Society. 2013;**135**:16120-16132

[34] Piccardo A, Paparo F, Puntoni M, Righi S, Bottoni G, Bacigalupo L, et al. 64CuCl2 PET/CT in prostate cancer relapse. Journal of Nuclear Medicine. 2018;**59**:444-451

[35] Ferrari C, Niccoli Asabella A, Villano C, Giacobbi B, Coccetti D, Panichelli P, et al. Copper-64 dichloride as theranostic agent for glioblastoma multiforme: A preclinical study. BioMed Research International. Hindawi Publishing Corporation. 2015;**2015**:6. Article ID 129764. DOI: 10.1155/2015/129764

[36] Jing X, Yang F, Shao C, Wei K, Xie M, Shen H, et al. Role of hypoxia in cancer therapy by regulating the tumor microenvironment. Molecular Cancer. 2019;**18**:1-15

[37] Sørensen BS, Horsman MR. Tumor hypoxia: Impact on radiation therapy and molecular pathways. Frontiers in Oncology. 2020;**10**:562

[38] Wong R, Fyles A, Milosevic M, Pintilie M, Hill RP. Heterogeneity of polarographic oxygen tension measurements in cervix cancer: An evaluation of within and between tumor variability, probe position, and track depth. International Journal of Radiation Oncology, Biology, Physics. 1997;**39**:405-412

[39] Lyng H, Malinen E. Hypoxia in cervical cancer: From biology to imaging. Clinical and Translational Imaging. 2017;**5**:373-388

[40] Matsumoto K-I, Szajek L, Krishna MC, Cook JA, Seidel J, Grimes K, et al. The influence of tumor oxygenation on hypoxia imaging in murine squamous cell carcinoma using [64Cu] Cu-ATSM or [18F] Fluoromisonidazole positron emission tomography. International Journal of Oncology. 2007;**30**:873-881

[41] Nie X, Elvington A, Laforest R, Zheng J, Voller TF, Zayed MA, et al. 64Cu-ATSM positron emission tomography/magnetic resonance imaging of hypoxia in human atherosclerosis. Circulation: Cardiovascular Imaging. 2020;**13**:e009791

[42] Liu J, Hajibeigi A, Ren G, Lin M, Siyambalapitiyage W, Liu Z, et al. Retention of the radiotracers 64Cu-ATSM and 64Cu-PTSM in human and murine tumors is influenced by MDR1 protein expression. Journal of Nuclear Medicine. 2009;**50**:1332-1339

[43] Fujibayashi Y, Taniuchi H, Yonekura Y, Ohtani H. Copper-62-ATSM: A new hypoxia imaging agent with high membrane permeability and low

redox potential. The Journal of Nuclear Medicine. 1997;**38**:1155

[44] Fujibayashi Y, Cutler C, Anderson C, McCarthy D, Jones L, Sharp T, et al. Comparative studies of Cu-64-ATSM and C-11-acetate in an acute myocardial infarction model: Ex vivo imaging of hypoxia in rats. Nuclear Medicine and Biology. 1999;**26**:117-121

[45] Dearling JL, Blower PJ. Redox-active metal complexes for imaging hypoxic tissues: Structure–activity relationships in copper (II) bis (thiosemicarbazone) complexes. Chemical Communications. 1998;(22):2531-2532. DOI: 10.1039/a805957h

[46] Tanaka T, Furukawa T, Fujieda S, Kasamatsu S, Yonekura Y, Fujibayashi Y. Double-tracer autoradiography with Cu-ATSM/FDG and immuno-histochemical interpretation in four different mouse implanted tumor models. Nuclear Medicine and Biology. 2006;**33**:743-750

[47] Yuan H, Schroeder T, Bowsher JE, Hedlund LW, Wong T, Dewhirst MW. Intertumoral differences in hypoxia selectivity of the PET imaging agent 64Cu (II)-diacetyl-bis (N4-methylthiosemicarbazone). Journal of Nuclear Medicine. 2006;**47**:989-998

[48] Dence CS, Ponde DE, Welch MJ, Lewis JS. Autoradiographic and small-animal PET comparisons between 18F-FMISO, 18F-FDG, 18F-FLT and the hypoxic selective 64Cu-ATSM in a rodent model of cancer. Nuclear Medicine and Biology. 2008;**35**:713-720

[49] Holland JP, Barnard PJ, Collison D, Dilworth JR, Edge R, Green JC, et al. Spectroelectrochemicalandcomputational studies on the mechanism of hypoxia selectivity of copper radiopharmaceuticals. Chemistry–A European Journal. 2008;**14**:5890-5907

[50] Liu T, Karlsen M, Karlberg AM, Redalen KR. Hypoxia imaging and theranostic potential of [64 Cu] [Cu (ATSM)] and ionic Cu (II) salts: A review of current evidence and discussion of the retention mechanisms. EJNMMI Research. 2020;**10**:1-14

[51] Lewis JS, McCarthy DW, McCarthy TJ, Fujibayashi Y, Welch MJ. Evaluation of 64Cu-ATSM in vitro and in vivo in a hypoxic tumor model. Journal of Nuclear Medicine. 1999;**40**:177-183

[52] Lapi SE, Lewis JS, Dehdashti F. Evaluation of hypoxia with copper-labeled diacetyl-bis (N-methylthiosemicarbazone). In: Seminars in Nuclear Medicine. Elsevier; 2015. pp. 177-185

[53] Colombié M, Gouard S, Frindel M, Vidal A, Chérel M, Kraeber-Bodéré F, et al. Focus on the controversial aspects of 64Cu-ATSM in tumoral hypoxia mapping by PET imaging. Frontiers in Medicine. 2015;**2**:58

[54] Lewis JS, Laforest R, Dehdashti F, Grigsby PW, Welch MJ, Siegel BA. An imaging comparison of 64Cu-ATSM and 60Cu-ATSM in cancer of the uterine cervix. Journal of Nuclear Medicine. 2008;**49**:1177-1182

[55] Anderson CJ, Ferdani R. Copper-64 radiopharmaceuticals for PET imaging of cancer: Advances in preclinical and clinical research. Cancer Biotherapy and Radiopharmaceuticals. 2009;**24**:379-393

[56] Gangemi V, Mignogna C, Guzzi G, Lavano A, Bongarzone S, Cascini GL, et al. Impact of [64 Cu] [Cu (ATSM)] PET/CT in the evaluation of hypoxia in a patient with glioblastoma: A case report. BMC Cancer. 2019;**19**:1-4

[57] Bourgeois M, Rajerison H, Guerard F, Mougin-Degraef M, Barbet J, Michel N, et al. Contribution of [64Cu]-ATSM PET

in molecular imaging of tumour hypoxia compared to classical [18F]-MISO—A selected review. Nuclear Medicine Review. 2011;**14**:90-95

[58] Dehdashti F, Mintun MA, Lewis JS, Bradley J, Govindan R, Laforest R, et al. In vivo assessment of tumor hypoxia in lung cancer with 60 Cu-ATSM. European Journal of Nuclear Medicine and Molecular Imaging. 2003;**30**:844-850

[59] Lopci E, Grizzi F, Russo C, Toschi L, Grassi I, Cicoria G, et al. Early and delayed evaluation of solid tumours with 64Cu-ATSM PET/CT: A pilot study on semiquantitative and computer-aided fractal geometry analysis. Nuclear Medicine Communications. 2017;**38**:340-346

[60] Grassi I, Nanni C, Cicoria G, Blasi C, Bunkheila F, Lopci E, et al. Usefulness of 64Cu-ATSM in head and neck cancer: A preliminary prospective study. Clinical Nuclear Medicine. 2014;**39**:e59-e63

[61] Vahidfar N, Farzanefar S, Ahmadzadehfar H, Molloy EN, Eppard E. A review of nuclear medicine approaches in the diagnosis and the treatment of gynecological malignancies. Cancers. 2022;**14**:1779

[62] Hueting R. Radiocopper for the imaging of copper metabolism. Journal of Labelled Compounds and Radiopharmaceuticals. 2014;**57**:231-238

[63] Mortimer JE, Kruper L, Cianfrocca M, Lavasani S, Liu S, Tank-Patel N, et al. Use of HER2-directed therapy in metastatic breast cancer and how community physicians collaborate to improve care. Journal of Clinical Medicine. 2020;**9**:1984

[64] Arienti C, Pignatta S, Tesei A. Epidermal growth factor receptor family and its role in gastric cancer. Frontiers in Oncology. 2019;**9**:1308

[65] Hayes DF. HER2 and breast cancer—A phenomenal success story. New England Journal of Medicine. 2019;**381**:1284-1286

[66] Slamon DJ, Clark GM, Wong SG, Levin WJ, Ullrich A, McGuire WL. Human breast cancer: Correlation of relapse and survival with amplification of the HER-2/neu oncogene. Science. 1987;**235**:177-182

[67] Press MF, Pike MC, Chazin VR, Hung G, Udove JA, Markowicz M, et al. Her-2/neu expression in node-negative breast cancer: Direct tissue quantitation by computerized image analysis and association of overexpression with increased risk of recurrent disease. Cancer Research. 1993;**53**:4960-4970

[68] Giordano SH, Temin S, Chandarlapaty S, Crews JR, Esteva FJ, Kirshner JJ, et al. Systemic therapy for patients with advanced human epidermal growth factor receptor 2–positive breast cancer: ASCO clinical practice guideline update. Journal of Clinical Oncology. 2018;**36**:2736-2740

[69] Jarrett AM, Hormuth DA, Adhikarla V, Sahoo P, Abler D, Tumyan L, et al. Towards integration of 64Cu-DOTA-trastuzumab PET-CT and MRI with mathematical modeling to predict response to neoadjuvant therapy in HER2+ breast cancer. Scientific Reports. 2020;**10**:1-14

[70] Kurihara H, Hamada A, Yoshida M, Shimma S, Hashimoto J, Yonemori K, et al. 64Cu-DOTA-trastuzumab PET imaging and HER2 specificity of brain metastases in HER2-positive breast cancer patients. EJNMMI Research. 2015;**5**:1-8

[71] Tamura K, Kurihara H, Yonemori K, Tsuda H, Suzuki J, Kono Y, et al. 64Cu-DOTA-trastuzumab PET imaging in patients with HER2-positive

breast cancer. Journal of Nuclear Medicine. 2013;**54**:1869-1875

[72] Bang Y-J, Van Cutsem E, Feyereislova A, Chung HC, Shen L, Sawaki A, et al. Trastuzumab in combination with chemotherapy versus chemotherapy alone for treatment of HER2-positive advanced gastric or gastro-oesophageal junction cancer (ToGA): A phase 3, open-label, randomised controlled trial. The Lancet. 2010;**376**:687-697

[73] Guo X, Zhu H, Zhou N, Chen Z, Liu T, Liu F, et al. Noninvasive detection of HER2 expression in gastric cancer by 64Cu-NOTA-trastuzumab in PDX mouse model and in patients. Molecular Pharmaceutics. 2018;**15**:5174-5182

[74] Chopra A. 64Cu-labeled DOTA-conjugated rituximab, a chimeric murine/human anti-CD20 monoclonal antibody. In: Molecular Imaging and Contrast Agent Database (MICAD) [Internet]. NLM, Bethesda: National Center for Biotechnology Information; 2012

[75] Natarajan A, Arksey N, Iagaru A, Chin FT, Gambhir SS. Validation of 64Cu-DOTA-rituximab injection preparation under good manufacturing practices: A PET tracer for imaging of B-cell non-Hodgkin lymphoma. Molecular Imaging. 2015;**14**. DOI: 10.2310/7290.2014.00055. PMID: 25762106

[76] Natarajan A, Gowrishankar G, Nielsen CH, Wang S, Iagaru A, Goris ML, et al. Positron emission tomography of 64Cu-DOTA-Rituximab in a transgenic mouse model expressing human CD20 for clinical translation to image NHL. Molecular Imaging and Biology. 2012;**14**:608-616

[77] James ML, Hoehne A, Mayer AT, Lechtenberg K, Moreno M, Gowrishankar G, et al. Imaging B cells in a mouse model of multiple sclerosis using 64Cu-rituximab PET. Journal of Nuclear Medicine. 2017;**58**:1845-1851

[78] Johnbeck CB, Knigge U, Loft A, Berthelsen AK, Mortensen J, Oturai P, et al. Head-to-head comparison of 64Cu-DOTATATE and 68Ga-DOTATOC PET/CT: A prospective study of 59 patients with neuroendocrine tumors. Journal of Nuclear Medicine. 2017;**58**:451-457

[79] Malmberg C, Ripa RS, Johnbeck CB, Knigge U, Langer SW, Mortensen J, et al. 64Cu-DOTATATE for noninvasive assessment of atherosclerosis in large arteries and its correlation with risk factors: Head-to-head comparison with 68Ga-DOTATOC in 60 patients. Journal of Nuclear Medicine. 2015;**56**:1895-1900

[80] Delpassand ES, Ranganathan D, Wagh N, Shafie A, Gaber A, Abbasi A, et al. 64Cu-DOTATATE PET/CT for imaging patients with known or suspected somatostatin receptor–positive neuroendocrine tumors: Results of the first US prospective, reader-masked clinical trial. Journal of Nuclear Medicine. 2020;**61**:890-896

[81] Carlsen EA, Johnbeck CB, Binderup T, Loft M, Pfeifer A, Mortensen J, et al. 64Cu-DOTATATE PET/CT and prediction of overall and progression-free survival in patients with neuroendocrine neoplasms. Journal of Nuclear Medicine. 2020;**61**:1491-1497

[82] de Camargo Etchebehere ECS, de Oliveira SA, Gumz B, Vicente A, Hoff PG, Corradi G, et al. 68Ga-DOTATATE PET/CT, 99mTc-HYNIC-octreotide SPECT/CT, and whole-body MR imaging in detection of neuroendocrine tumors: A prospective trial. Journal of Nuclear Medicine. 2014;**55**:1598-1604

[83] Bodei L, Ambrosini V, Herrmann K, Modlin I. Current concepts in

68Ga-DOTATATE imaging of neuroendocrine neoplasms: Interpretation, biodistribution, dosimetry, and molecular strategies. Journal of Nuclear Medicine. 2017;**58**:1718-1726

[84] Pfeifer A, Knigge U, Binderup T, Mortensen J, Oturai P, Loft A, et al. 64Cu-DOTATATE PET for neuroendocrine tumors: A prospective head-to-head comparison with 111In-DTPA-octreotide in 112 patients. Journal of Nuclear Medicine. 2015;**56**:847-854

[85] Hicks RJ, Jackson P, Kong G, Ware RE, Hofman MS, Pattison DA, et al. 64Cu-SARTATE PET imaging of patients with neuroendocrine tumors demonstrates high tumor uptake and retention, potentially allowing prospective dosimetry for peptide receptor radionuclide therapy. Journal of Nuclear Medicine. 2019;**60**:777-785

[86] Johnbeck CB, Knigge U, Kjær A. PET tracers for somatostatin receptor imaging of neuroendocrine tumors: Current status and review of the literature. Future Oncology. 2014;**10**:2259-2277

[87] Mirzaei S, Revheim M-E, Raynor W, Zehetner W, Knoll P, Zandieh S, et al. 64Cu-DOTATOC PET-CT in patients with neuroendocrine tumors. Oncology and Therapy. 2020;**8**:125-131

[88] Vahidfar N, Fallahpoor M, Farzanehfar S, Divband G, Ahmadzadehfar H. Historical review of pharmacological development and dosimetry of PSMA-based theranostics for prostate cancer. Journal of Radioanalytical and Nuclear Chemistry. 2019;**322**:237-248

[89] Calabria F, Pichler R, Leporace M, Wolfsgruber J, Coscarelli P, Dunzinger A, et al. 68Ga/64Cu PSMA bio-distribution in prostate cancer patients: Potential pitfalls for different tracers. Current Radiopharmaceuticals. 2019;**12**:238-246

[90] Vali R, Loidl W, Pirich C, Langesteger W, Beheshti M. Imaging of prostate cancer with PET/CT using 18F-Fluorocholine. American Journal of Nuclear Medicine and Molecular Imaging. 2015;**5**:96

[91] Morris MJ, Akhurst T, Osman I, Nunez R, Macapinlac H, Siedlecki K, et al. Fluorinated deoxyglucose positron emission tomography imaging in progressive metastatic prostate cancer. Urology. 2002;**59**:913-918

[92] Sanz G, Robles J, Gimenez M, Arocena J, Sanchez D, Rodriguez-Rubio F, et al. Positron emission tomography with 18fluorine-labelled deoxyglucose: Utility in localized and advanced prostate cancer. BJU International. 1999;**84**:1028-1031

[93] Minamimoto R, Uemura H, Sano F, Terao H, Nagashima Y, Yamanaka S, et al. The potential of FDG-PET/CT for detecting prostate cancer in patients with an elevated serum PSA level. Annals of Nuclear Medicine. 2011;**25**:21-27

[94] Effert P, Beniers A, Tamimi Y, Handt S, Jakse G. Expression of glucose transporter 1 (Glut-1) in cell lines and clinical specimens from human prostate adenocarcinoma. Anticancer Research. 2004;**24**:3057-3064

[95] Shiiba M, Ishihara K, Kimura G, Kuwako T, Yoshihara N, Sato H, et al. Evaluation of primary prostate cancer using 11C-methionine-PET/CT and 18F-FDG-PET/CT. Annals of Nuclear Medicine. 2012;**26**:138-145

[96] Kennedy EP, Weiss SB. The function of cytidine coenzymes in the biosynthesis of phospholipides. Journal of Biological Chemistry. 1956;**222**:193-214

[97] Wang Y, Kent C. Effects of altered phosphorylation sites on the properties of CTP: Phosphocholine cytidylyltransferase. Journal of Biological Chemistry. 1995;**270**:17843-17849

[98] Beheshti M, Imamovic L, Broinger G, Vali R, Waldenberger P, Stoiber F, et al. 18F choline PET/CT in the preoperative staging of prostate cancer in patients with intermediate or high risk of extracapsular disease: A prospective study of 130 patients. Radiology. 2010;**254**:925-933

[99] Chondrogiannis S, Marzola MC, Grassetto G, Maffione AM, Rampin L, Veronese E, et al. New acquisition protocol of 18F-choline PET/CT in prostate cancer patients: Review of the literature about methodology and proposal of standardization. BioMed Research International. 2014;**2014**. DOI: 10.1155/2014/215650. PMID: 25121090; PMCID: PMC4119889

[100] Hodolic M. Role of 18F-choline PET/CT in evaluation of patients with prostate carcinoma. Radiology and Oncology. 2011;**45**:17

[101] Cantiello F, Crocerossa F, Russo GI, Gangemi V, Ferro M, Vartolomei MD, et al. Comparison between 64Cu-PSMA-617 PET/CT and 18F-choline PET/CT imaging in early diagnosis of prostate cancer biochemical recurrence. Clinical Genitourinary Cancer. 2018;**16**:385-391

[102] Grubmüller B, Baum RP, Capasso E, Singh A, Ahmadi Y, Knoll P, et al. 64Cu-PSMA-617 PET/CT imaging of prostate adenocarcinoma: First in-human studies. Cancer Biotherapy and Radiopharmaceuticals. 2016;**31**:277-286

[103] Capasso E, Durzu S, Piras S, Zandieh S, Knoll P, Haug A, et al. Role of 64CuCl2 PET/CT in staging of prostate cancer. Annals of Nuclear Medicine. 2015;**29**:482-488

[104] Sparks R, Peng F. Positron emission tomography of altered copper metabolism for metabolic imaging and personalized therapy of prostate cancer. Journal of Radiology and Radiation Therapy. 2013;**1**:1015

[105] Hoberück S, Wunderlich G, Michler E, Hölscher T, Walther M, Seppelt D, et al. Dual-time-point 64 Cu-PSMA-617-PET/CT in patients suffering from prostate cancer. Journal of Labelled Compounds and Radiopharmaceuticals. 2019;**62**:523-532

[106] Cantiello F, Gangemi V, Cascini GL, Calabria F, Moschini M, Ferro M, et al. Diagnostic accuracy of 64copper prostate-specific membrane antigen positron emission tomography/ computed tomography for primary lymph node staging of intermediate-to high-risk prostate cancer: Our preliminary experience. Urology. 2017;**106**:139-145

[107] Woo S-K, Jang SJ, Seo M-J, Park JH, Kim BS, Kim EJ, et al. Development of 64Cu-NOTA-trastuzumab for HER2 targeting: A radiopharmaceutical with improved pharmacokinetics for human studies. Journal of Nuclear Medicine. 2019;**60**:26-33

[108] Liu T, Liu C, Zhang Z, Zhang N, Guo X, Xia L, et al. 64Cu-PSMA-BCH: A new radiotracer for delayed PET imaging of prostate cancer. European Journal of Nuclear Medicine and Molecular Imaging. 2021;**48**:4508-4516

[109] Pfeifer A, Knigge U, Mortensen J, Oturai P, Berthelsen AK, Loft A, et al. Clinical PET of neuroendocrine tumors using 64Cu-DOTATATE: First-in-humans study. Journal of Nuclear Medicine. 2012;**53**:1207-1215

[110] Matias M, Pinho JO, Penetra MJ, Campos G, Reis CP, Gaspar MM. The

challenging melanoma landscape: From early drug discovery to clinical approval. Cell. 2021;**10**:3088

[111] Anderson CJ, Dehdashti F, Cutler PD, Schwarz SW, Laforest R, Bass LA, et al. 64Cu-TETA-octreotide as a PET imaging agent for patients with neuroendocrine tumors. Journal of Nuclear Medicine. 2001;**42**:213-221

[112] Persson M, Skovgaard D, Brandt-Larsen M, Christensen C, Madsen J, Nielsen CH, et al. First-in-human uPAR PET: Imaging of cancer aggressiveness. Theranostics. 2015;**5**:1303

[113] Ahrens BJ, Li L, Ciminera AK, Chea J, Poku E, Bading JR, et al. Diagnostic PET imaging of mammary microcalcifications using 64Cu-DOTA-alendronate in a rat model of breast cancer. Journal of Nuclear Medicine. 2017;**58**:1373-1379

[114] Avila-Rodriguez M, Rios C, Carrasco-Hernandez J, Manrique-Arias J, Martinez-Hernandez R, Garcia-Perez F, et al. Biodistribution and radiation dosimetry of [64Cu] copper dichloride: First-in-human study in healthy volunteers. EJNMMI Research. 2017;**7**:1-7

[115] Laforest R, Dehdashti F, Lewis JS, Schwarz SW. Dosimetry of 60/61/62/64Cu-ATSM: A hypoxia imaging agent for PET. European Journal of Nuclear Medicine and Molecular Imaging. 2005;**32**:764-770

Chapter 6

Radiochemical Purity and Identity in Radiopharmaceuticals: Design and Improvement of Quality Control Methods by HPLC

Roberto Mercado, Silvia Lagos and Ethel Velásquez

Abstract

The radiopharmaceutical supply chain involves rigorous quality control tests to assure products are safe and effective to use in the clinic. However, one of the key challenges for analytical methods in radiopharmacy is the narrow time frame where the analysis must be completed due to the limited half-life of radiomolecules. Radiochemical purity and identity are critical tests to control the success of radiolabeling. These parameters are easily determined by thin-layer chromatography methods (TLC) in some widely used molecules such as [^{18}F]FDG. However, for new diagnostic and therapeutic agents with more complex radiolabeling steps, it is critical to have better separations to identify impurity peaks only detectable using higher sensitive methods. This chapter will present the keys to designing and improving high-performance liquid chromatography (HPLC) methods for radiopharmaceutical analysis, with practical examples of method optimization. It will also be reviewed how to determine the main parameters necessary for the validation of an analytical method, and finally, some approaches to the use of liquid chromatography coupled with mass detectors in tandem (LC-MS/MS) during the development of radiopharmaceuticals will be presented.

Keywords: quality control, radiopharmaceuticals, supply chains, improvements, pharmaceutical, production

1. Introduction

Radiopharmaceuticals are medicinal products that contain radionuclides and are used for diagnostic and therapeutic purposes. In view of such products being intended for use in humans and the fact that they are generally administered intravenously to the patient, it is essential to ensure product quality from the beginning of the manufacturing phase within the supply chain. Therefore, quality control tests that include sampling, physicochemical and microbiological tests of raw materials and finished products are an essential part of quality assurance. Modern and specific regulations for radiopharmaceuticals mention that laboratory analytical methods must be suitable for their intended use, meaning they must be sensitive, specific, precise, and reproducible [1, 2].

Quality control analysis for radiopharmaceuticals include some simple methods, such as a visual inspection to ensure that their appearance is a clean, transparent solution without particulate matter. It is also necessary to measure the pH of injectable solutions, which can be done easily with a pH meter or a pH paper strip, through the use of a minimal aliquot to perform the measurement. Other analyses aim to identify the unique presence of the desired radioisotope by calculating its half-life and radionuclidic purity using gamma spectroscopy. However, the determination of radiochemical purity (RCP), chemical purity (CP), and the identity of a radiopharmaceutical are of particular interest to evaluate the quality of radiolabeling.

1.1 Radiochemical purity

Radiochemical purity of the radiopharmaceutical preparation can be defined as the proportion of the radionuclide activity present in the indicated chemical form (A_{RPh}). As shown in eq. 1, radiochemical purity is expressed as a percentage relative to the total radioactive species in the sample (A_T)

$$\%RCP = \frac{A_{RPh}}{A_{Total}} * 100 \tag{1}$$

Since the radiochemical form of the radiopharmaceutical determines its biochemical behavior, it is necessary to control radiochemical impurities that may alter the desired biodistribution and modify specific uptake, subsequently affecting the diagnostic image or treatment being administered. Radiochemical impurities can originate from changes that occur during storage and deviations that occur during the production process of the radioisotope or radiopharmaceutical. The generation of radiochemical impurities can also derive from the radiolysis process of the radiolabeled molecule, originating fragments that contain the radiation-emitting isotope. In order to be detected, a process of separation of the radiochemical impurities is required; chromatographic separation and analysis methods are most suitable for determining radiochemical purity [3].

1.2 Chemical purity

The determination of chemical purity aims to detect and quantify those chemical impurities that may affect the quality of radiolabeling or generate adverse reactions in patients. These impurities are nonradioactive compounds that can be generated during radiolabeling as synthesis by-products, residues from a precursor, or auxiliary raw materials used in some steps of the production process, such as residual solvents. They can also be intentionally added substances such as stabilizers to delay radiolysis or other types of additives. In some cases, the presence of these impurities is unavoidable, so they must be controlled to a maximum value present in the preparation, which is usually declared in the product monographs. Due to the different nature of these impurities, it is necessary to evaluate the use of various techniques depending on the type of analyte. For example, residual solvents used during the synthesis process such as acetonitrile, dimethyl sulfoxide, or ethanol are detected by gas

DOI: http://dx.doi.org/10.5772/intechopen.112355

chromatography. Others, such as Kryptofix 2.2.2 or tetrabutylammonium carbonate, are detected by a spot test revealed with resublimated iodine. However, impurities related to reaction by-products or remnants of precursors usually have a similar structure and polarities to the radiopharmaceutical, then requiring methods with greater separation capacity such as high-performance liquid chromatography [3].

1.3 Identity

The identity of the radiopharmaceutical refers to the verification of the presence of the radiopharmaceutical within the mixture. This verification is performed by analyzing a nonradioactive standard (cold standard) solved in a similar matrix to the radiopharmaceutical sample. In this way, the coincidence of the retention time (t_r) or retention factor (R_f) between the cold standard and the radiopharmaceutical unequivocally identifies the presence of the compound of interest.

2. Separation techniques used in radiopharmacy

During the radiopharmacy practice, the most commonly used techniques for determining identity, radiochemical purity, and chemical purity are thin-layer chromatography (TLC) and high-performance liquid chromatography (HPLC).

2.1 Thin-layer chromatography

This technique is a form of solid-liquid chromatography where the stationary phase is usually a polar absorbent thin-layer and a liquid mobile phase that can be a solvent or a mixture of them. Analysis of radiopharmaceuticals by thin-layer chromatography is performed by depositing a few microliters of the analyte onto a plate containing finely ground silica (e.g. TLC Silica Gel 60 plates), Whatman cellulose chromatography paper (e.g. Whatman 1 CHR) or glass microfiber chromatography paper (e.g. iTLC-SG), which is then placed on a plate or impregnated on fiberglass. This plate with the sample is placed in a chamber containing the mobile phase. The solvent, which is at the bottom of the chamber, moves up the adsorbent layer by capillary action and passes over the point where the sample was seeded; as it continues upward, the solvent moves the compounds in the mixture up the plate at different rates. The result is the separation of compounds due to differences in their affinity with the stationary phase and differences in solvent solubility [4].

Once the solvent has run to the front mark, the plate is removed and visualized using ultraviolet light, iodine, or sulfuric acid solution. In contrast, for radiopharmaceutical products a dedicated instrument radio-TLC scanner is required, such as the Eckert & Ziegler/Bioscan model Mini-Scan radio-TLC scanner, which is shown in **Figure 1**, Panel A. This type of equipment is commonly used in routine quality control of radiopharmaceuticals such as [^{18}F]FDG and [^{99m}Tc]$NaTcO_4$ [5, 6]. It has a detector containing a counting gas (9:1 Argon:Methane) and an electrode; when the chromatographic run is finished, the TLC plate is placed in the equipment, and then the detector moves over the surface at an appropriate speed to optimize the count. The control software records the count as the detector moves to obtain the radiochromatogram [5]. Other manufacturers of these instruments are Elysia-Raytest, Capintec, Scannix and Lablogic. **Figure 1**, Panel B shows a radio-TLC chromatogram of [^{99m}Tc]$NaTcO_4$ sample. A retention factor (R_f) ranging from 0.7 to 1 identifies the

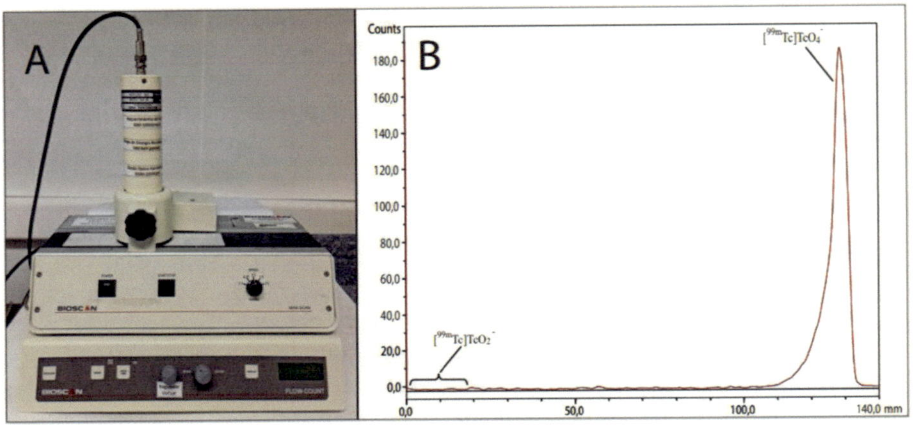

Figure 1.
(Panel A) Eckert & Ziegler/bioscan radio-TLC scanner, mini-scan model. (Panel B) radio-TLC chromatogram of [^{99m}Tc]$NaTcO_4$ sample.

pertechnetate [$^{99m}TcO_4$]$^-$ species, while an R_f between 0 and 0.1 identifies reduced/hydrolyzed species [$^{99m}TcO_2$]$^-$.

Using this simple technique, it is also possible to perform identity and radiochemical purity assays on radiocompounds. This is carried out by performing a test in parallel with the radiopharmaceutical analysis; to this aim, a drop of cold standard of the radiopharmaceutical is tested, being eluted with a selected mobile phase according to the polarity of the analyte and compatible with the stationary phase present on the TLC plate. This cold standard can be visualized by ultraviolet light (UV) or revealed by resublimated iodine, while the plate bearing the radiopharmaceutical sample is read on a radio-TLC scanner. The radiochemical purity is quantified by the percentage of peak area related to the total sample, while the radiochemical identity is confirmed by comparing the retention factor (R_f) of the radiochemical peak with that of the unmarked standard. To determine the identity and radiochemical purity of these compounds, it is necessary that the implemented method ensures that there is no co-elution of the analytes and provides different retention factors for each of them. One way to achieve this purpose is to use different mobile phase systems with suitable polarity for each analyte to be separated. It is for this reason that several mobile phases with the same stationary phase present in the chromatographic support are frequently used to perform a single analysis of radiochemical purity, chemical purity, or identity by TLC.

It is also possible to perform radiochemical purity analysis using TLC by manually cutting the chromatographic strip into several equal parts and then measuring them individually using a dose calibrator or an automated gamma counter. This alternative is especially useful when the laboratory does not have a radio-TLC scanner. However, this method of measurement is not the most suitable due to several disadvantages, mainly:

- High variability in the radiochemical purity assessment, which is related to how uniformly the pieces have been cut.

- If the cut segments are too large, there is a risk of overlooking some chromatographic peaks.

- Due to the geometry of the detector, the measurement can be affected by the position of the strip section relative to the detector.

- The high manipulation required by the analyst to perform the measurement in this way can introduce errors in the result.

- Cutting and measuring the chromatographic strips carries the risk of cross-contamination between samples.

- The time it takes to individually measure each piece of the chromatographic strip makes it very slow compared to using a radio-TLC scanner.

2.2 High-performance liquid chromatography

HPLC is an evolution of TLC, which offers better separation capacity by injecting a radiopharmaceutical sample into a packed liquid chromatography column, where its components are separated based on their polarity while being eluted by a suitable mobile phase. Due to the chemical and physical composition of the chromatographic column and the composition of the mobile phase used, this system can achieve better separations than thin-layer chromatography, even when the sample contains substances with similar polarities.

This instrument has a pump that propels the mobile phase at a sufficient pressure to travel through the packed column, eluting the sample through it. Once the sample has been separated, it can be detected by different types of detectors depending on the type of analyte to be analyzed. In the case of radiopharmaceuticals, a UV detector senses the chromophores of the sample, and a radiometric detector determines the gamma radiation emitted by the radioisotope linked to the radiopharmaceutical are commonly used. Similarly to TLC, it is possible to identify the radiopharmaceutical using a cold standard [3], this time by the coincidence of the retention time. In addition, having a quantitative detector like the UV, it is possible to identify and quantify the radiopharmaceutical and its impurities, which gives it a significant advantage over less quantitative methods such as TLC. Other detectors with more limited use in radiopharmacy are the refractive index detector, due to its lower sensitivity compared to UV detectors, and the pulsed amperometric detector, as the radiomolecules to be measured must be electroactive [7].

Figure 2 shows an Agilent 1190 radiochromatograph, which has a quaternary pump that allows manipulation of up to four solvents to form the mobile phase, and diode array detector (DAD) that measures the absorbance of the sample throughout the UV-Visible spectrum while performing the chromatographic run, providing an advantage in the development of quantitative analysis methods. Finally, this equipment has a NaI crystal Raytest radiation detector connected in series that allows radiometric measurements when the analyte has radioactive properties.

2.3 TLC versus HPLC in radiopharmacy

Several factors should be evaluated to select between TLC and HPLC such as the analytes to be analyzed, equipment and resource availability, sensitivity and precision requirements, or research objectives to get the proper quality control method as part of the supply chain or in an R&D radiopharmaceutical environment. It is important to consider that the choice between TLC and HPLC may vary depending on the specific

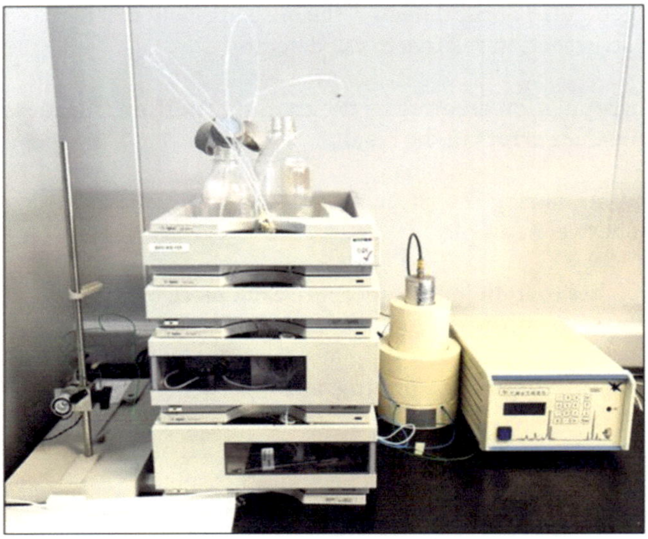

Figure 2.
Radio-HPLC system with diode array detector and radiometric detector. Some manufacturers of these instruments are Agilent, Dionex, Shimadzu, waters, among others.

requirements of the radiopharmaceutical and the available capabilities. **Table 1** summarizes some advantages and disadvantages of TLC and HPLC.

3. Recommendations for the development of measurement methods in HPLC liquid chromatography for radiopharmaceuticals

Many times, setting an analysis method for a novel radiopharmaceutical or a radiopharmaceutical already on the market seems to be a very extensive job, especially when it comes to the development of an HPLC method or any other instrumental technique. The development of HPLC methods not only involves determining the instrumental parameters that will be used but also involves creating a complete procedure that will guide the analyst through the assay. Therefore, it is very important to identify the purpose of the analytical method to be developed, which in this case is multiple, since as previously mentioned, using liquid chromatography, it is possible to verify the identity of the radiopharmaceutical and also determine its chemical and radiochemical purity.

3.1 Initial steps

To initiate the HPLC method development process, it is very important to collect background information and data about the analyte to be measured, which include conducting a review of the literature to obtain some initial conditions for an analysis to be optimized, or estimate its polarity and other attributes as chromophore groups that help select an analytical separation column and mobile phase. During this stage, it is also advisable to fully understand the radiolabeling reaction and to have a chemical criterion when proposing the identity of unknown impurities that may be found during the analysis. At the same time, in the case of PET radiopharmaceuticals, it is

Attribute	TLC	HPLC
Simplicity and speed of analysis	Quick and simple analysis	Requires more preparation and analysis is usually slower
Cost	Economic analysis. The cost of TLC plates is affordable. Lower solvent consumption	Chromatographic columns are more expensive than TLC plates. Higher consumption of solvents.
Method validation	Method validation with TLC is generally easier.	More complex validation
Analyte limitations	Few limitations regarding the nature of the analyte.	Colloidal species and aggregates are not detected as they are retained at the top of the column.
Separation capacity	Low separation capacity	High separation capacity for analytes with similar polarities. Suitable for analysis of impurities generated by radiolysis.
Sensibility	Poor sensitivity. Limited impurity detection capacity.	HPLC detectors have a higher sensitivity and allow impurity quantification.
Versatility of the technique	Few optimization options.	Method optimization can be reached by modifying mobile phase gradients, injection volume, dimensions and column composition, among others.
Simultaneous analysis	Several chromatographic runs on different mobile phases are necessary to separate different compounds from a sample	It is possible to determine chemical purity, radiochemical purity, and identity with just one chromatographic run.
Automation	Very few automation options	A wide variety of autosamplers allows automatic analysis optimizing time in the laboratory.

Table 1.
Comparison between some attributes of TLC and HPLC. Advantages in green.

important to test a sample of the synthesis precursor with the developed method. This way it is possible to identify chemical and radiochemical impurities based on the retention time (t_r) and thus classify these compounds as a known impurity.

3.2 Column selection

To obtain successful chromatography, an adequate balance is required between the intermolecular forces existing between the three active participants in the separation process: the solute, the mobile phase, and the stationary phase. These intermolecular forces are qualitatively described in terms of the relative polarity of each of the three reactants. In general, the polarity in increasing order for various functional groups present in the analyte is: hydrocarbons < ethers < esters < ketones < aldehydes < amides < amines < alcohols. Water is more polar than any compound containing some of the above functional groups [8].

Since radiopharmaceuticals are usually radiolabeled variants of other better-known molecules such as hormones, sugars, nucleosides, or peptides, it is recommended to conduct a literature search for analysis methods for the original molecule in order to select a column. A special consideration should be given related to the behavior of the radiopharmaceutical which can be slightly different due to the modifications in its structure. For example, in the case of fluorinated radiopharmaceuticals, the strong electronegativity of fluorine makes these compounds slightly more lipophilic, increasing their retention time compared to their nonfluorinated analog, while the behavior in radiopharmaceuticals labeled with metals such as technetium-99 m also tends to increase due to the necessary use of bifunctional chelating agents for their radiolabeling, which can change the lipophilicity of the molecule.

In addition to the composition of the stationary phase, another parameter to consider is the column dimension and physical characteristics of its packed particles, which can affect chromatographic separation. A 250 mm column will have good separation capacity, but it will increase analysis time. Therefore, it is recommended to choose shorter columns that also decrease the size of the packing particles. For example, a column with the same C18 phase and chromatographic conditions of 250 mm and a particle size of 5 μm will have separation efficiency similar to a C18 column of 150 mm and 2.6 μm. However, since the analyte has to travel a shorter distance, the analysis will be faster, which is particularly important in short-lived radiopharmaceuticals such as those labeled with fluorine-18 or carbon-11. **Figure 3** shows the injection of a standard solution of OH-PSMA and cold-standard of [^{18}F]PSMA-1007 at a concentration of 10 μg/mL in a 250 mm C18 column with a particle size of 5 μm (Panel A) and the same sample in a 150 mm C18 column with a particle size of 2.6 μm (Panel B). It is possible to observe how the change in dimensions alone reduces the retention time of both analytes and the total time of the chromatographic run.

It is possible to observe the use of this strategy in the recent monograph of the European Pharmacopeia for [^{18}F]PSMA-1007 [9], in which the method described by Cardinale et al. [10] for determining the chemical purity of this radiopharmaceutical was optimized. The cost of this improvement will be the increase in instrument pressure, so it is suggested to monitor that the pressure does not exceed 80% of the maximum pressure supported by the system in order to not decrease its useful life.

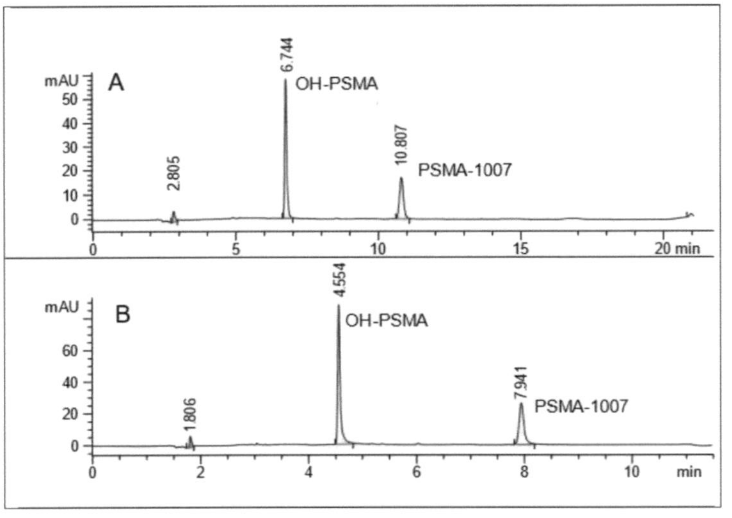

Figure 3.
Comparison of two columns with the same C18 stationary phase. Panel a has dimensions of 250 x 4.6 mm x 5 μm, and panel B has dimensions of 150 x 4.6 mm x 2.6 μm.

In addition to the packed columns previously described, there are other kinds of columns called monolithic columns. Monolith technology can be imagined as a single porous "particle" filling the entire volume of the column without any of the interparticle spaces typical of packed columns. This forces the mobile phase to circulate completely through the stationary phase. Silica monolithic columns are characterized by higher porosities than packed particle columns, with greater column efficiency, higher permeability, and, consequently, they allow for working with a higher flow of mobile phase. However, not everything is advantageous, as higher porosity implies a lower amount of silica in the column, which will lead to less stationary phase after the corresponding chemical modification (which provides functionality to the column). This will result in lower retention for analytes [11].

In the case of radiopharmaceuticals, monolithic columns can be useful when packed columns easily saturate and present a tailing effect. If saturation occurs, there is also a risk of radioactive material accumulation within the column, increasing exposure to the analyst who handles the instrument, which can be avoided with the use of a monolithic column. In **Figure 4**, Panel A shows the chromatogram of a sample of a peptide HYNIC-iPSMA using a C18 column of 150 x 4.6 mm, with a particle size of 2.7 µm and a pore size of 165 Å. Saturation of the column or two overlapping chromatographic peaks can be observed. Chromatogram in Panel B shows the same sample, with the same chromatographic conditions, but using a C18 monolithic column of 100 x 4.6 mm, with a mesopore size of 13 nm and macropores of 2 µm. At least two chromatographic peaks can be observed that were previously overlapped with the previous column.

3.3 Selection of mobile phase

As mentioned in the previous section, it is recommended to perform a literature search for analysis methods of the original molecule, in order to have guidance on the mobile phase to be used. In many reverse-phase separations, a solvent mixture of water and a polar organic solvent such as acetonitrile, methanol or ethanol is

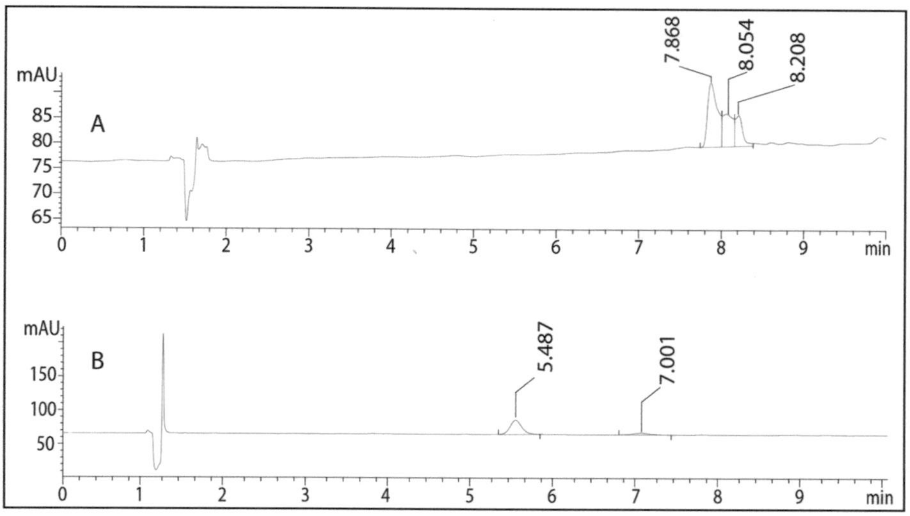

Figure 4.
Chromatographic analysis of the precursor peptide HYNIC-iPSMA.

employed. The retention time of the analyte can be manipulated by varying the water concentration. For example, in a C8 stationary phase column with a mobile phase composed of acetonitrile and water, the retention of steroids increases with increasing water proportion, improving the analysis resolution [8].

In analyses using ultraviolet absorption as a detection method, it is important to consider that each solvent has its own specific absorbance cut-off wavelength. Below this wavelength, the solvent itself absorbs the light. When choosing a solvent, its limit and where the desired analytes will absorb should be considered. If the analyte wavelengths are close, a different solvent should be chosen. The following list shows the UV cut-off wavelengths of some of the most used liquid chromatography solvents (**Table 2**).

3.4 Selection of detection wavelength

Most radiopharmaceuticals analyzed by RP-HPLC contain chromophore groups that are detected with UV-Visible detectors. Therefore, it is convenient to identify the wavelength of maximum absorption of the analyte to maximize the sensitivity of the method under construction. For this purpose, the best option is to have a diode array detector (DAD) that allows analyzing the absorbance spectrum of each chromatographic peak separated by the analysis column.

In radiopharmaceuticals such as [^{18}F]FES, (recently approved by FDA like Cerianna), where the limited amount administered is only 5 μg per patient injection, it is important to have a method with high sensitivity [12, 13]. **Figure 5** shows the absorbance spectrum of a sample of the radiopharmaceutical [^{18}F]FES obtained with

Solvent	λ (Cut-off) [nm]
Acetonitrile	190
Water	191
Heptane	197
Ciclohexane	210
Ethanol	210
Methanol	210
Hexane	210
2-propanol	210
Tetrahydrofuran	220
Chloroform	245
Ethyl acetate	255
Dimethylsulfoxide	264
Toluene	286
Acetic acid	260
Acetone	330

Table 2.
Cut-off of the most used solvents in liquid chromatography.

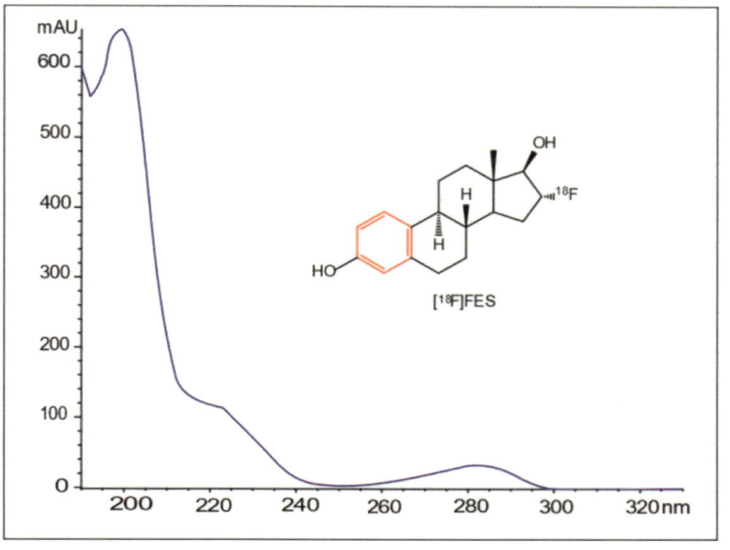

Figure 5.
[18F]FES absorption spectrum obtained by liquid chromatography using a diode array detector.

a diode array detector. In the represented structure, the main chromophore can be observed in red as the aromatic ring in conjugation. Although the absorption region between 260 and 290 nm may be more selective and some authors use it for quantification [14–17], it is possible to increase the sensitivity of the method by using the band from 225 to 235 nm, taking care not to approach the cut-off zone of the solvents used in the mobile phase.

3.5 Consider the effect of the matrix

During the development of the chromatographic method, it is important to know the matrix of the finished product, as it could act as an interferent during the HPLC analysis, either by a change in the sample pH shifting retention times, or a difference in pH between the mobile phase and the sample containing buffer salts, which could cause the crystallization of these salts inside the HPLC system, obstructing the equipment and generating complications during the analysis. In the synthesis of PET radiopharmaceuticals, sodium ascorbate or citrate buffer solutions are commonly used to regulate the final solution pH to around 7. Therefore, the presence of these salts should be considered during the chromatographic method development.

For example, the effect of the matrix can be observed in the last step of the synthesis of [^{18}F]PSMA-1007, where 400 mg of sodium ascorbate is added with the purpose of reducing the radiation-induced degradation that becomes noticeable in activities produced above 20 GBq [10]. **Figure 6**, Panel A shows the chromatogram of an injection of freshly synthesized [^{18}F]PSMA-1007 without the presence of ascorbic acid, where it is easy to visualize [^{18}F]PSMA-1007 and its impurities. Meanwhile, the chromatogram of **Figure 6**, Panel B shows a sample of a new synthesis with sodium ascorbate at a concentration of 20 mg/mL, where a large peak of sodium ascorbate can be appreciated, which masks the analytes that need to be quantified.

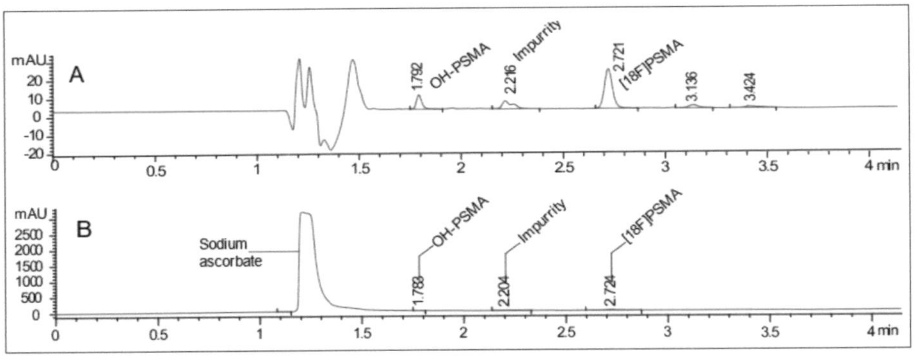

Figure 6.
Matrix effect of sodium ascorbate in a [^{18}F]PSMA-1007 synthesis sample.

4. Aspects to consider in the validation of methods for radiopharmaceuticals in HPLC

The validation of an analytical method aims to establish by means of scientific studies that a method is suitable for its intended use. In validation, some analytical properties or characteristics of the method that account for its reliability to be applied are determined. One of the most used guidelines for validation is produced by the International Conference of Harmonization of Technical Requirements for Registration of Pharmaceuticals for Human Use and Validation of Analytical Procedures, Text, and Methodology [18] and considers the study of the following analytical properties for method validation. Additionally, the European Association of Nuclear Medicine provides a validation guide focused on the validation of radio-analytical methods used in the quality control of radiopharmaceuticals [2].

4.1 Determination of the linearity or determination range

This corresponds to the most reliable concentration range for measuring the analyte. This range is between the concentration corresponding to the method's limit of quantification and the maximum concentration delivered by the limit of linearity. In the case of radiopharmaceuticals, the specifications are usually provided as a maximum injectable mass for a patient in a maximum injection volume (Vmax), which will result in a maximum allowable concentration (Cmax). This Vmax volume is defined by the radiopharmaceutical producer and may depend on its presentation (single-dose syringes or multi-dose vials). When a calibration curve is constructed, Cmax should be at the center of the calibration curve, since, in the linear regression model, the least uncertainty is found at the center of the calibration curve.

To illustrate, the radiopharmaceutical [^{18}F]PSMA-1007 has a maximum injectable limit of 100 μg per patient injection. In this case, it has been defined that Vmax will be 5 mL, resulting in a Cmax of 20 μg/mL. Therefore, a calibration curve was constructed that includes points 5, 10, 20, 30, and 40 μg/mL, where six replicates were injected to build the calibration curve, as shown in **Figure 7**.

Visually, the data fit the linear model, and its Pearson's R coefficient value is 0.9980. However, none of these criteria is conclusive to ensure the linearity of the method. To ensure that the data fits the linear model, it is suggested to perform a Lack of Fit test in some statistical software [19]. Since it is a hypothesis test, for the example in **Figure 7**,

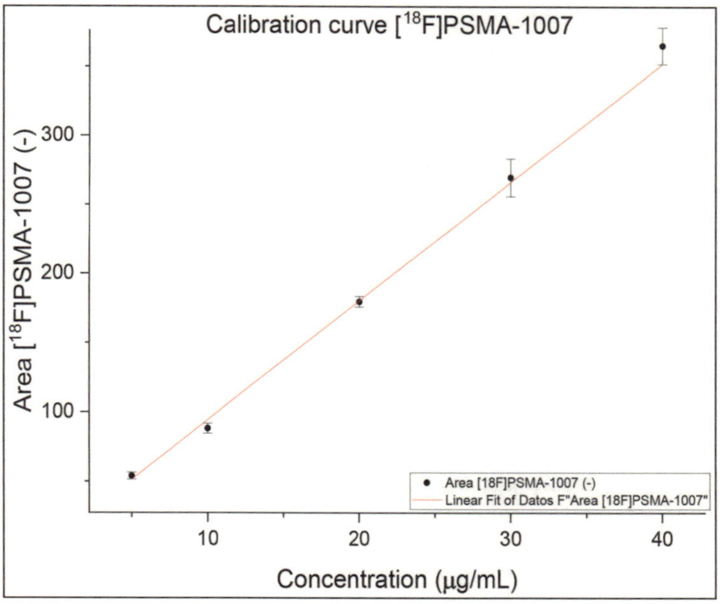

Figure 7.
Calibration curve for [^{18}F]PSMA-1007.

the p-value obtained for this data was 0.5135; given that this p-value>0.05, then there is no evidence against the null hypothesis, and it can be concluded that the linear model is appropriate for modeling the calibration data for [^{18}F]PSMA-1007.

4.2 Selectivity

Specificity or selectivity is the ability of an analytical method to measure an analyte accurately and specifically without interference from impurities, degradation products, additives, or coproducts. A chromatographic method is specific if it can separate the component of interest from other components in the formulation [3]. Using the example of the chromatographic analysis of [^{18}F]PSMA-1007 in **Figure 6**, Panel A, it is possible to verify the separation of each of the sample's components.

The separation of the individual components of the sample demonstrates the method's selectivity. To do so, it is necessary to inject each component of the sample beforehand to determine its retention time and, therefore, its elution order. During the development of an analytical method and once the elution order has been established, it is important not to make significant changes to the chromatographic method that involve drastic polarity changes (such as changing the solvent of the mobile phase or column), as this can change the elution order of the sample's components.

4.3 Precision

Precision is the degree of agreement among a group of results and is represented as the dispersion of these results around their mean. Precision is usually expressed as variance, standard deviation, or coefficient of variation (CV) of a series of measurements. In the case of detecting impurities with a standard solution, such as OH-PSMA in the synthesis of [^{18}F]PSMA-1007, multiple analyses of OH-PSMA at different concentrations within the previously determined linear range are necessary. A CV value less than 10% demonstrates the precision of the method [3].

4.4 Accuracy

Accuracy expresses the closeness between the accepted value as the reference value (certified reference material) and the found value (average value) obtained by applying the analysis procedure a certain number of times. Accuracy is usually expressed in terms of relative error.

To properly determine the accuracy of a measurement in a chemical purity analysis by HPLC in radiopharmaceuticals, it is essential to have certified reference material for impurities and a cold standard of the radiopharmaceutical. Usually, in the chemical purity analysis of PET radiopharmaceuticals, the criterion is used that impurities have the same molar extinction coefficient as the radiopharmaceutical. This criterion is an approximation based on the assumption that the precursor used has a high degree of purity, that the synthesis coproducts are structurally similar, and that the chromophoric groups have not degraded. Despite the widespread use of this practice, from a strictly analytical point of view, it is an error because it does not use a certified reference material for each impurity. Finally, in multistep syntheses where more than one synthesis precursor is used, it is more complex to make this approximation, as it is more likely that one of the precursors does not have the same molar extinction coefficient as the main analyte.

4.5 Robustness

It is the ability of a method to not be affected by small, intentionally made changes in method parameters. An HPLC method is considered robust when the results are not affected by small variations in mobile phase pH, mobile phase composition, flow rate, or changes in supplier or batch of the separation columns used [3].

4.6 Recovery

Sometimes, certain precursor radioisotopes of the radiopharmaceutical (e.g., [^{18}F]Fluoride or [^{99m}Tc]$NaTcO_4$) can become retained in the HPLC injection system, tubing, precolumn, or column [2]. To evaluate the recovery, the two simplest methods to perform are:

- Compare the injected activity with the eluted activity by collecting eluted fractions and measuring them with a dose calibrator.
- Remove the column and precolumn and perform a second chromatographic run, comparing the peak areas of the two chromatograms while correcting for decay. However, this method does not take into account the activity that may be retained by the tubing or the injector.

4.7 Calculation of detection and quantification limits

There are different ways to calculate the detection limit (LOD), defined as the lowest amount of analyte detectable, and the quantification limit (LOQ), defined as the lowest amount of analyte quantifiable. One of the ways to calculate the LOD and LOQ of a method according to statistical criteria is based on the ratio between the magnitude of the measurement signal and the background noise produced by the instrument or the analytical blank. For example, the detection limit defined by IUPAC is the concentration of analyte that produces a signal that can be statistically differentiated from an analytical blank and is calculated by measuring the response of at least ten independent analytical blanks from which the mean (Yb) and standard deviation (σ_b) are determined. According to IUPAC, the detection limit is:

$$Y_{LD} = Y_b + 3\sigma_b \tag{2}$$

A concentration C_{LD} corresponds to a signal Y_{LD}, which is achieved by graphic extrapolation on the calibration curve.

Despite the simplicity of calculating the limit of detection using the IUPAC methodology, its application in liquid chromatography is challenging, as determining the blank area value requires selecting a region of the chromatogram corresponding to the analyte's retention time (radiopharmaceutical) that corresponds to the baseline without any apparent signal. Therefore, a practical way to calculate the limit of detection and quantification is to prepare a calibration curve with concentrations below the last point on the calibration curve with at least three points and six replicates at each level [20]. Then, to calculate the LOD and LOQ using Eqs. (3) and (4), respectively, where S_a is the standard deviation of the intercept at low concentrations, a is the intercept of the low concentration curve, b is the slope of the calibration curve at high concentrations, and n is the number of replicates.

$$LOD = \frac{|a| + 3S_a}{b * \sqrt{n}} \tag{3}$$

$$LOQ = \frac{|a| + 10S_a}{b * \sqrt{n}} \tag{4}$$

5. The frontier: Use of liquid chromatography coupled to mass detectors in radiopharmaceuticals

Liquid chromatography coupled to mass detectors (LC-MS) is an analytical technique that involves the chromatographic separation of analytes, followed by their detection based on mass spectrometry. Although its use is relatively new, its sensitivity, selectivity, and precision have made it a technique of choice for detecting quantities of micrograms or even nanograms in a sample. This high sensitivity can be interesting in the analysis of radiopharmaceuticals due to the low quantities of radioactive molecules present in the formulations.

Unlike HPLC with UV detectors, as mentioned above, in LC-MS, the mobile phase carrying the separated analytes is not allowed to reach the mass spectrometer. While a conventional HPLC system operates at ambient pressures, the mass spectrometer operates under vacuum, and both systems (HPLC and MS) are coupled through an interface. During an analysis, the mobile phase elutes through the column toward the interface, the solvent is evaporated with heat, and the analyte molecules are vaporized and ionized. This is a crucial step since the mass spectrometer is only capable of detecting and measuring the ions in the gas phase. Since the analyte ions are generated at atmospheric pressure in the interface, the process is called atmospheric pressure ionization (API), and the interface is known as an API ion source. Electrospray ionization (ESI), electron ionization (EI), and matrix-assisted laser desorption/ionization (MALDI) are the most used ionization sources in LC-MS analysis.

In such a detector, analyte ions are introduced into the mass spectrometer, where they are subjected to electric and/or magnetic fields. The flight paths of the ions are altered by varying the applied fields, ensuring their separation from one another based on their mass-to-charge values, m/Z. After separation, the ions can be collected and detected by a variety of mass detectors, where the most common analyzer is the quadrupole type. It is possible to couple two mass analyzers that function in series, which allows for the precise identification and quantification of different types of samples. These triple quadrupole QQQ or TQMS (Triple Quadrupole Mass Spectrometer) and quadrupole time-of-flight QTOF mass spectrometers are the most commonly used tandem mass detectors. The combination of liquid chromatography (LC) with tandem mass detectors (MS/MS) gives rise to LC-MS/MS.

Figure 8 shows a working scheme of a triple quadrupole detector, where the sample gets to an ionization source after being separated in the HPLC system. For samples with medium to high polarity and high molecular weights, an ESI source is commonly used. Once the sample is ionized, it is separated in the first quadrupole (Q1), and one of the produced ions is selected and further fragmented in the second quadrupole (Q2), which is used as a collision cell to obtain new fragments. These are then selected in the third quadrupole (Q3) and finally detected at the end of the spectrometer.

In the field of radiopharmacy, in radiolabeling processes that involve complex chemical synthesis, impurities are usually produced, some of which can be identified by the coincidence of the retention time with a reference standard for such impurities or they may be residues of the precursor. However, the identity of other impurities that normally occur in very low quantities can only be classified as a coproduct. Their quantification is approximated by assuming that they have the same molar extinction coefficient as the analyte of interest [10, 17], and their chemical structure can only be speculated through careful analysis of the reaction. LC-MS/MS is a technique that provides complementary information for the identification of these impurities since, together with the separation provided by the chromatographic column, tandem analyzers can provide the fragmentation patterns of the components of the sample, which help to elucidate the structure of these impurities and quantify them.

On the other hand, LC-MS/MS has been used to characterize and evaluate the specific activity of rapidly decaying radiopharmaceuticals such as those using

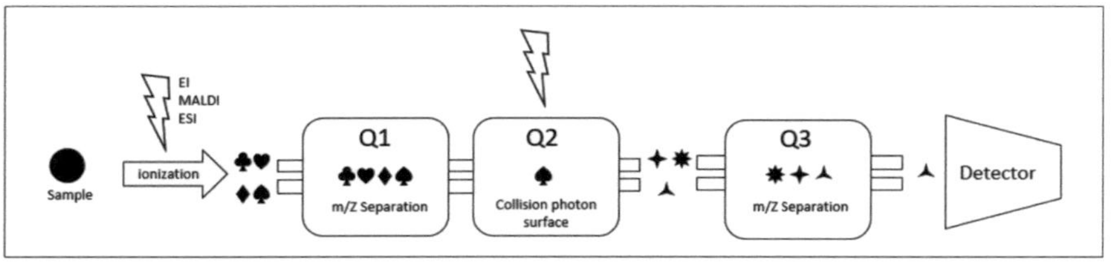

Figure 8.
Operating diagram of a triple quadrupole mass spectrometer TQ or QqQ.

carbon-11 [21]. Specific activity is the ratio between the amount of a compound (mol) in radioactive and nonradioactive form (isotopologues) at a specific time when the measurement is made. The precise determination of specific activity is critical in radiocompounds that will bind to low-density protein targets such as neurotransmitter receptors, enzymes, or in specific cases where the radiopharmaceutical is pharmacologically very potent, such as dopamine, nicotinic, or opioid receptor radiotracers [21–24].

Usually, in routine practice, this measurement is made using HPLC systems with UV detectors coupled to a radiometric detector. However, the accuracy of these detectors is vulnerable to errors in instrumental settings. LC-MS/MS has been demonstrated to be an autonomous, rapid, and reliable tool for measuring specific activity in radiocompounds present in trace amounts by tracking the radiolabeled fragments while also identifying the position of radiolabeling in the prepared tracer.

6. Conclusions

Currently, in routine radiopharmaceutical practice, thin-layer chromatography (TLC) and the use of a radio-TLC scanner are the gold standard for evaluating the radiochemical purity in radiopharmaceuticals. This is due to the simplicity of the technique, low solvent consumption, and its robustness. With this technique and the use of a cold standard, it is also possible to determine the identity and chemical purity of a radiopharmaceutical using developers such as ultraviolet light, sublimated iodine, or sulfuric acid. However, the separation capacity of chromatographic plates and the sensitivity of the developers used are not always convenient for determining impurities present in radiopharmaceuticals. On the other hand, as the development of radiopharmaceuticals aims at molecules that interact with specific biological targets and the synthesis processes become more complex, generating coproducts with similar polarities to the radiopharmaceutical. Therefore, it is necessary to use a technique with better separation capacity, such as high-performance liquid chromatography (HPLC). With the appropriate choice of mobile phase, a separation column that considers the physicochemical properties of the analyte, and a detection wavelength that maximizes method sensitivity, it is possible to separate and quantify the target analyte from its impurities even though they have similar polarities. By adding the use of a cold standard, it is possible to determine the identity of a radiopharmaceutical, and due to the superior separation and detection capacity of HPLC, it is possible to visualize coproducts and other impurities that are present at low concentration levels.

From a quality assurance standpoint, it is necessary to verify that analytical methods that use TLC or HPLC for the determination of radiochemical purity, identity, and chemical purity have the conditions to generate accurate and reproducible results through validation of the method. The validation process includes the evaluation of linearity, selectivity, precision, accuracy, robustness, and calculation of the limit of detection and quantification. Validation should include detailed documentation of the analysis method and procedures used for sample preparation, as well as the training and qualification of personnel performing the analysis.

In the field of radiopharmaceutical research, it is possible to use chromatographs that are coupled to mass spectrometers that are used as detectors. An LC-MS/MS can be used for the identification and quantification of compounds based on their mass-to-charge ratio (m/Z). By identifying and quantifying charged analyte fragments produced in a tandem mass detector, it is possible to obtain structural information on impurities produced during a radiolabeling reaction. It should be noted that a triple quadrupole mass detector itself is not a suitable tool for determining the complete structure of a molecule; theoretical knowledge of the radiolabeling reaction is required beforehand to have a chemical criterion for proposing an analyte structure. In order to elucidate a structure, it is convenient to combine LC-MS/MS with other techniques such as nuclear magnetic resonance spectroscopy (NMR), infrared spectroscopy (IR), and molecular modeling provided by computational chemistry. On the other hand, in some specific cases, it is possible to use a triple quadrupole mass detector as a complementary tool to determine the radiochemical purity of a radiopharmaceutical. For example, if the mass of the radioactive fragment of interest is known and radioactive impurities with different masses are suspected, a triple quadrupole mass detector could help identify and quantify impurities in the sample.

Conflict of interest

The authors declare no conflict of interest.

Appendices and nomenclature

TLC	thin-layer chromatography
[^{18}F]FDG	2-deoxy-2-[18F]fluoroglucose
HPLC	high-performance liquid chromatography
RP-HPLC	reversed-phase high-performance liquid chromatography
LC-MS	liquid chromatography-mass spectrometry
LC-MS/MS	liquid chromatography coupled with Mass detectors in tandem
RCP	radiochemical purity
CP	chemical purity
Rf	retention factor
t_r	retention time
UV	ultraviolet light
PET	Positron emission tomography
^{99m}Tc	Technetium-99 m
[^{99m}Tc]$NaTcO_4$	[^{99m}Tc] Sodium pertechnetate
C18	Octadecylsilane
C8	Octylsilane
OH-PSMA	Hydroxy-PSMA-1007; 2-{3-[1-Carboxy-5-(2-{4-[(4-carboxy-2-{4-carboxy-2-[(6-oxo-1,6-dihydro-pyridine-3-carbonyl)-amino]-butyrylamino}-butyrylamino)-methyl]-benzoylamino}-3-naphthalen-2-yl-propionylamino)-pentyl]-ureido}-pentanedioic acid
[^{18}F]PSMA-1007	18-Fluorine-PSMA-1007; (3S,10S,14S)-1-(4-(((S)-4-carboxy-2-((S)-4-carboxy-2-(6-[18F]fluoronicotinamido)butanamido)butanamido)methyl)phenyl)-3-(naphthalen-2-ylmethyl)-1,4,12-trioxo-2,5,11,13-tetraazahexadecane-10,14,16-tricarboxylic acid
HYNIC	hydrazinonicotinic acid
HYNIC-iPSMA	HYNIC-Lys(Nal)-urea-Glu
[^{18}F]FES	16α-[^{18}F]-fluoro-17β-fluoroestradiol; (8S,9S,13S,16R,17R)-16-[^{18}F]fluoro-13,17-dimethyl-7,8,9,11,12,13,14,15,16,17-decahydro-6H-cyclopenta[a]phenanthren-3-ol
Vmax	maximum volume

Cmax	maximum concentration
CV	coefficient of variation
EANM	European Association of Nuclear Medicine
LOD	limit of detection
LOQ	limit of quantification
IUPAC	International Union of Pure and Applied Chemistry
API	atmospheric pressure ionization
ESI	electrospray ionization
EI	electron ionization
MALDI	matrix-assisted laser desorption/ionization
TQMS or QQQ	triple quadrupole mass spectrometer
QTOF	quadrupole time-of-flight mass spectrometer

Author details

Roberto Mercado*, Silvia Lagos and Ethel Velásquez
Centro de Investigaciones Nucleares para Aplicaciones en Salud y Biomedicina (CINASB), División de Investigación y Aplicaciones Nucleares, Comisión Chilena de Energía Nuclear, Santiago, Chile

*Address all correspondence to: roberto.mercado@cchen.cl

References

[1] Current good manufacturing practice for positron emission tomography drugs. Federal Register. Food and Drug Administration. 2009;**74**:65409

[2] Gillings N, Todde S, Behe M, Decristoforo C, Elsinga P, Ferrari V, et al. EANM guideline on the validation of analytical methods for radiopharmaceuticals. EJNMMI Radiopharmacy and Chemistry. 2020;**5**(1):7. DOI: 10.1186/s41181-019-0086-z

[3] Lodi F, Boschi F. Quality control of PET radiopharmaceuticals. In: Khalil M, editor. Basic Science of PET Imaging. 1st ed. Cham: Springer; 2016. pp. 105-126. DOI: 10.1007/978-3-319-40070-9_5

[4] Skoog D, Holler J, Nieman T. Principios de Análisis Instrumental. 5th ed. Madrid: McGraw-Hill; 2001. p. 824

[5] USP 40 NF 35. Farmacopea de Estados Unidos. Fludesoxiglucosa F 18, Rockville: Inyección; 2017. pp. 4673-4675

[6] USP 38 NF 33. Farmacopea de los Estados Unidos. Pertecnetato de Sodio Tc 99m, Rockville: Inyección; 2015. pp. 5881-5882

[7] Thompson S, Scott P. Equipment and instrumentation for radiopharmaceutical chemistry. In: Lewis J, Windhorst A, Zeglis B, editors. Radiopharmaceutical Chemistry. 1st ed. Switzerland: Springer; 2019. pp. 481-499. DOI: 10.1007/978-3-319-98947-1_27

[8] Skoog D, Holler J, Nieman T. Principios de Analisis Instrumental. 5th ed. Madrid: McGraw-Hill; 2001. pp. 803-807

[9] European Pharmacopoeia (Ph. Eur.) Supplement 10.5. European Directorate for Quality of Medicines & Healthcare. Strasbourg: PSMA-1007 (18F) Injection; 2021. pp. 5725-5727

[10] Cardinale J, Martin R, Remde Y, Schäfer M, Hienzsch A, Hübner S, et al. Procedures for the GMP-compliant production and quality control of [^{18}F]PSMA-1007: A next generation Radiofluorinated tracer for the detection of prostate cancer. Pharmaceuticals [Internet]. 2017;**10**(4):77. DOI: 10.3390/ph10040077

[11] Nuñez O. Columnas monolíticas de base sílice: Propiedades, preparación, modificaciones químicas y aplicaciones en cromatografía de líquidos. Cromatografía y técnicas afines. 2008;**29**(2):59-77

[12] CERIANNA (Fluoroestradiol F 18) Injection, for Intravenous Use Initial U.S. Approval: 2020 [Internet]. Available from: https://www.accessdata.fda.gov/drugsatfda_docs/label/2020/212155s000lbl.pdf [Accessed: April 28, 2023]

[13] Updated Specifications for IND #79,005[F-18]FES [F-18]Fluoroestradiol [Internet]. Available from: https://imaging.cancer.gov/programs_resources/cancer-tracer-synthesis-resources/docs/FES_spec_sheet.pdf [Accessed: April 28, 2023]

[14] Kumar P, Mercer J, Doerkson C, Tonkin K, McEwan J. Clinical production, stability studies and PET imaging with 16-α-[18F]fluoroestradiol ([^{18}F]FES) in ER positive breast cancer patients. Journal of Pharmacy and Pharmaceutical Sciences. 2007;**10**(2):256-265

[15] Bispo A, Nascimento LTC, Costa FM, Da Silva JB, Mamede M. Development of an HPLC method for the radiochemical

purity evaluation of [^{18}F]fluoroestradiol. Brazilian Journal of Radiation Sciences. 2019;**7**(2A):01-09. DOI: 10.15392/bjrs.v7i2A.746

[16] Yilmaz B, Kadioglu Y. Determination of 17 β-estradiol in pharmaceutical preparation by UV spectrophotometry and high-performance liquid chromatography. Arabian Journal of Chemistry. 2017;**10**(1):S1422-S1428. DOI: 10.1016/j.arabjc.2013.04.018

[17] Oh SJ, Chi DY, Mosdzianowski C, Kil HS, Ryu JS, Moon DH. The automatic production of 16alpha-[^{18}F] fluoroestradiol using a conventional [18F]FDG module with a disposable cassette system. Applied Radiation and Isotopes. 2007;**65**(6):676-681. DOI: 10.1016/j.apradiso.2006.06.016

[18] International Conference of Harmonization of Technical Requirements for Registration of Pharmaceuticals for Human Use and Validation of Analytical Procedures, Text, and Methodology (ICH Q2R1). Nov 2005

[19] Brüggemann L, Quapp W, Wennrich R. Test for non-linearity concerning linear calibrated chemical measurements. Accreditation and Quality Assurance. 2006;**11**(12):625-631. DOI: 10.1007/s00769-006-0205-x. DOI: 10.1186/2191-219x-3-3

[20] Sanabri L, Marinez J, Baenay. Validación de una metodología analítica por HPLC-DAD para la cuantificación de cafeína en un ensayo de permeación in vitro empleando mucosa oral porcina. Revista Colombiana de Ciencias Químicas y Farmacéuticas. 2017;**46**(2):202-219

[21] Shetty HU, Morse CL, Zhang Y, Pike VW. Characterization of fast-decaying PET radiotracers solely through LC-MS/MS of constituent radioactive and carrier isotopologues. EJNMMI Research. 2013;**3**(3):1-8. DOI: 10.1186/2191-219x-3-3

[22] Kung M-P, Kung HF. Mass effect of injected dose in small rodent imaging by SPECT and PET. Nuclear Medicine and Biology. 2005;**32**:673-678. DOI: 10.1016/j.nucmedbio.2005.04.002

[23] Mizrahi R, Houle S, Vitcu I, Ng A, Wilson AA. Side effects profile in humans of (11)C-(+)-PHNO, a dopamine D(2/3) agonist ligand for PET. Journal of Nuclear Medicine. 2010;**51**(3):496-497. DOI: 10.2967/jnumed.109.072314

[24] Madsen K, Marner L, Haahr M, Gillings N, Knudsen GM. Mass dose effects and in vivo affinity in brain PET receptor studies--a study of cerebral 5-HT4 receptor binding with [^{11}C] SB207145. Nuclear Medicine and Biology. 2011;**38**(8):1085-1091. DOI: 10.1016/j.nucmedbio.2011.04.006